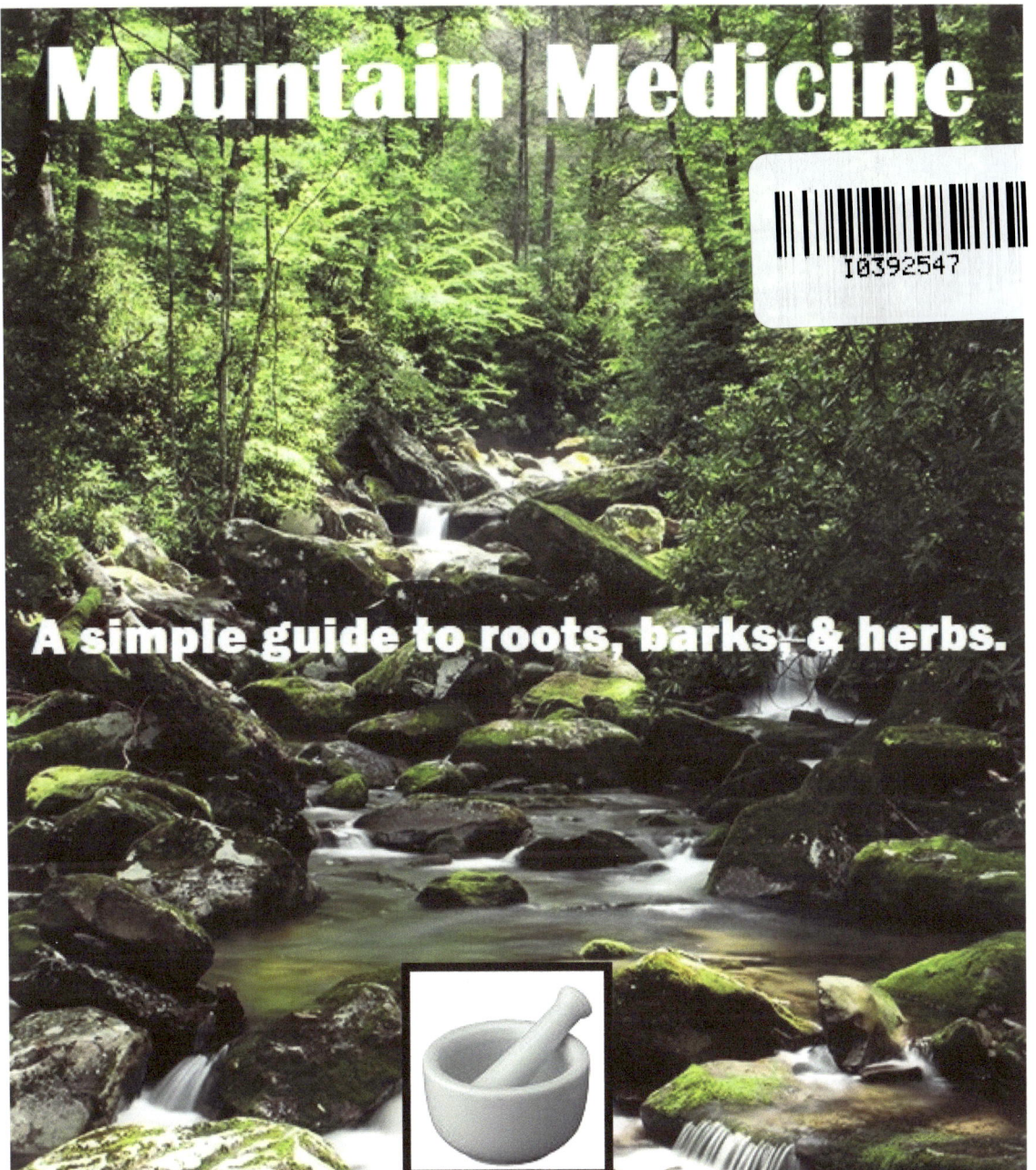

Mountain Medicine

A SIMPLE FIELD GUIDE TO PLANTS, ROOTS, BARKS, AND HERBS
COMMONLY FOUND IN APPALACHIA AND YOUR OWN BACK YARD.

This is a simple guide to plants, roots, barks, and herbs commonly found in the Appalachian Mountains and many places around the country. Growing up in Eastern Kentucky, I spent a lot of time in the forests with my parents and grandparents. They taught me the different kinds of plants and roots you could forage and gather to either make money with or make your home remedies. This guide is intended to educate readers on the identity of these plants, roots, and barks. It is also intended to give some idea of what they can be used for, and an estimate of their value. My family would make extra income by gathering and selling roots. This book is mainly intended as a guide for those who seek to do the same. While home remedies can be made from natural sources, this book is not intended to replace conventional medicines nor persuade anyone to do so. If you are sick, go to the doctor. That being said, you never know when the day may come when one might be in a situation where this knowledge might be to one's advantage. In this book you will find some of the most commonly sought plants and roots. All plants, roots, herbs, and barks should be dried naturally before use or sale. People who use natural remedies obtained from natural sources have had a lifetime of experience. I cannot stress enough that if you do not know what you are doing, then don't do it. You do so at your own risk. Also, I must talk about ownership. You own the wild plants and herbs on your property. If you seek to hunt on someone else's property, while most probably would not mind, you must get permission first. You cannot hunt on state or federally owned lands without written permission. People who break the laws and hunt on lands they do not own without permission can face serious fines and even imprisonment. Some things may be harvested in national parks and forests for personal use but may not be sold. Also, what and how much you may harvest varies depending on many factors. As a general rule, if you do not know then always ask first. Laws on what you may harvest and when you may harvest it also varies depending on your region. Always know the laws in your region first. For more information contact your local forestry division.

Table of Contents

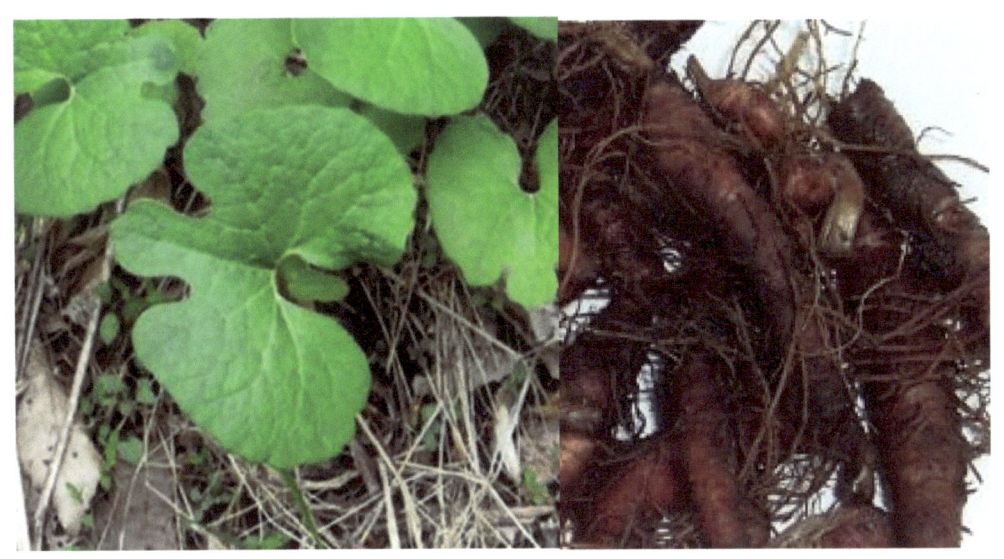

Blood Root

Sanguinaria Canadensis

Also known as "Coon Root" or "Red Root" because of its blood red color. While not as valuable as some roots you can find, it makes up for it in quantity. It is usually found in patches and is quite common and easy to find. Native Americans would use this root for dye and some medicines for skin conditions and stomach problems. It was also sometimes used for sore throat and cough, though used in large amounts it can induce vomiting. While sometimes the root was used in modern medicines for these same issues it is most commonly used in mouthwash and toothpaste. Like all roots, the price fluctuates but is usually worth anywhere between 4.00$ - 12.00$ a pound depending on current market demand.

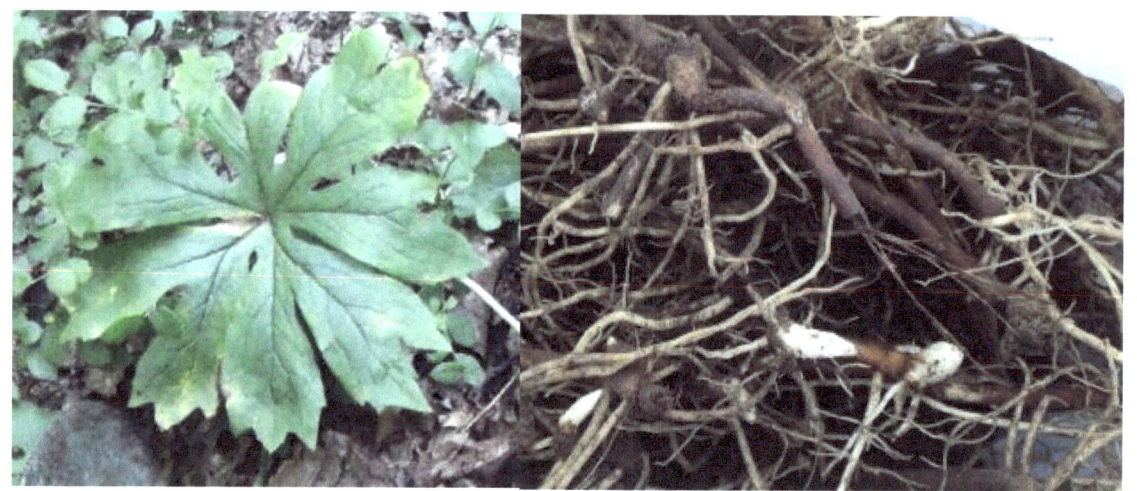

May Apple

Podophyllum Peltatum

Called May Apple, because in the month of May the plant will produce a small white flower that produces something resembling an apple. The apple is the only edible part of the plant. All other parts are considered poison. While also called yellow root by some, yellow root is known as a completely different plant in some regions. This is a very common plant and the value is not very much, but again if makes up for this in how common it is. It has been used a topical treatment for genital warts and hairy leukoplakia. May Apple is a relative of the Barberry and Golden Seal plant. The price varies with the market but is usually between 1.00$ - 3.00$ a pound to root buyers. You can find people selling it online these days for a lot more to people who seek natural roots and plants to make their own home remedies.

Barks are one of the things I want to include in this book. In recent years "barkers" have become a real problem in some areas. The bark of some trees have quite a bit of value to them and since trees tend to grow around others of their own kind, it makes them really easy to find. The problem is that these tress are usually on someone elses property. The way they harvest the bark is kind of ingenious. People will cut a ring around the bottoms of some trees and create slits around the tree. They will them use a knife or some tool to pry some of the bark off the tree. Some barks are really fiberous. Imagine a pack of bread ties. They are all attached to each other, like the bark of a tree. You pull the bottom of one of the ties and it peels away from the reast of the pack. Some barks are harvested in the same way. Once you have a piece of bark started to peel off the tree, you can pull it while walking away from the tree and pull a strip of bark off almost all the way to the top of the tree. You just go around the tree repeating this process until all the bark is removed from the tree. The problem is that this kills the tree if more than a quarter of the bark is removed. Thieves will go onto someone else's property and destroy whole groves of trees. It takes really no time to harvest an entire pickup truck full of tree bark and then sell it for a few hundred dollars. It is because when the bark is completely removed from a tree and the tree dies and can not regenerate the bark that makes the bark so valuable. While not valuable in small quantities, it is really easy to gather a large quantity at the risk of killing the tree....and going to jail if you are on someone else's property.

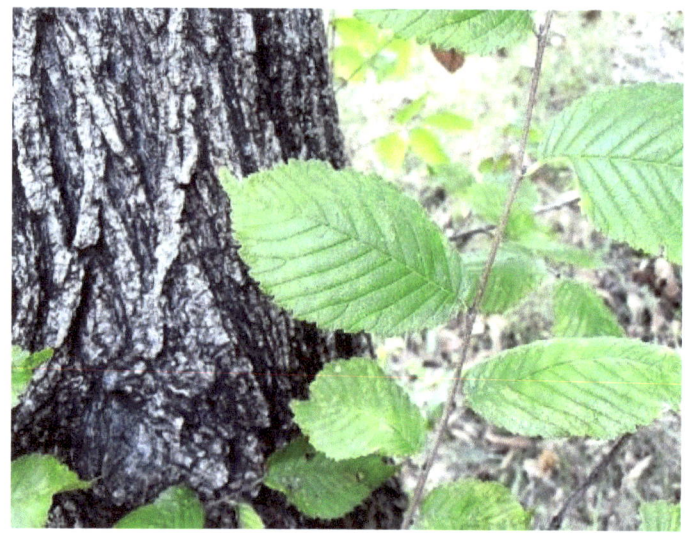

Slippery Elm (Bark)

Ulmas Rubra

Slippery Elm is harvested from the bark of a specific type of elm tree. This is something I have seen my grandmother use a lot. She would put the bark into a jar of water and leave it. Over time the water would turn into a clear looking slime that is really, well, slippery. Hence the name. She would use it as a topical ointment for various things, but it has been used by Native Americans as a medicine to treat anything from wounds to gastrointestinal ailments. To give you a more scientific explanation, slippery elm contains a type of soluble fiber known as mucilage. When placed in water the mucilage will trap and absorb the water. After some time, it will form a gel-like substance or slime that is slippery and can coat mucous membranes. It can provide short-term relief of pain and inflammation. It also contains a high calcium content may also be used as a mild antacid. The price of this varies from region to region and depends on the current market. It is widely sold as capsules and powders.

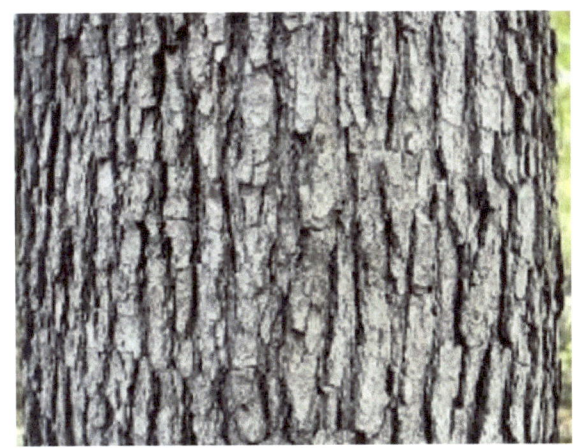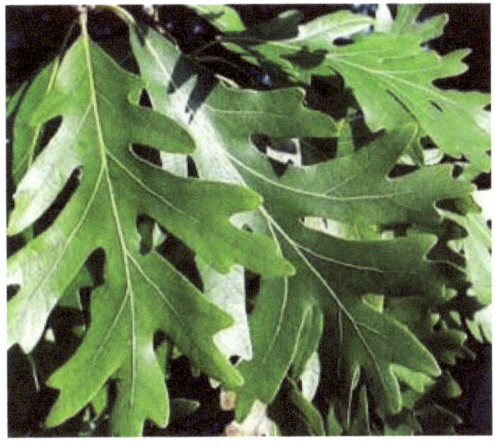

White Oak (Bark)

Quercus Alba

White Oak be recognized by the blunt lobes of its leaves. White oak bark can be boiled

into a tea and used for arthritis, diarrhea, colds, fever, cough, and bronchitis. It can also be

used used by people who want to increase their appetite and improve their digestion.

Some people use the it topically on the skin in a compress or bandage or use it in their

bath for a variety of pain and inflamation of the skin. Sometimes in the mouth, throat,

genital, or anal regions. The bark is regarded as a good source of iron and B-12. Again the

price varies depending on region and demand depending on the buyer. To give you an

idea of value, the people who buy it to resell can make 2.00$ an ouce or 7.50$ a pound for

white oak bark.

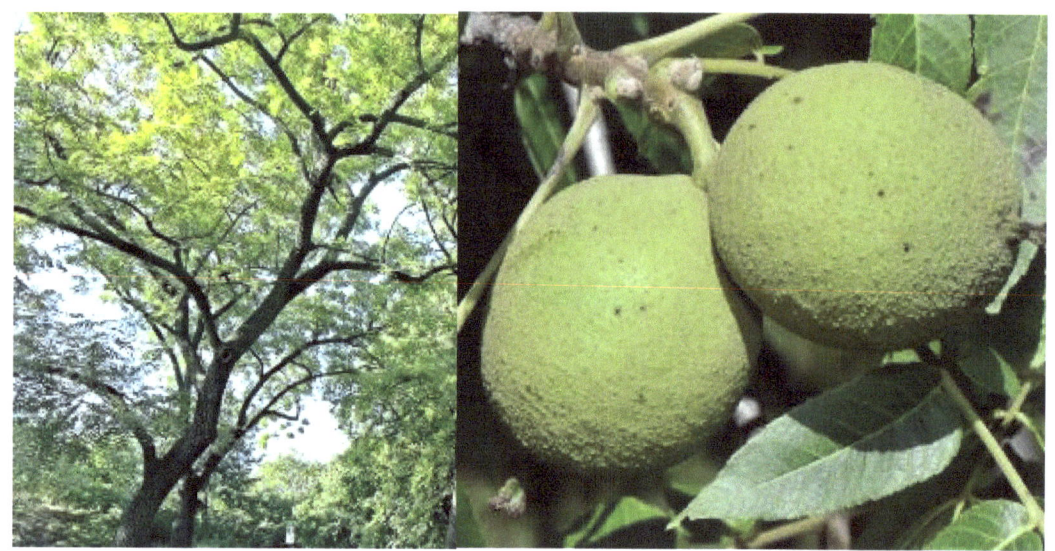

Black Walnut

Juglans Nigra

Black Walnut is harvested and used for its leaves and walnust hulls. Be warned, black walnut hulls can be very messy. Black Walnut leaves are usually harvested in the mid to late summer while the plant is in bloom. The hull of the nut itself can be used to make medicine for parasites and worms in the body. It can also be used to help with infections and syphilis. Though I would recommend going to the doctor and obtaining some penecilin. You can make penecilin yourself, though again I would recommend going to the doctor, but then you never know when the day may come when something happens and you can't go to the doctor. That is why it may be good to know this stuff besides just making some extra money. The hulls are really messy and some actually use it as a hair dye. While the nut can be eaten the price for all the parts you can sell fluctuates, but generally a pound of leaves will fetch you around a 1.50$.

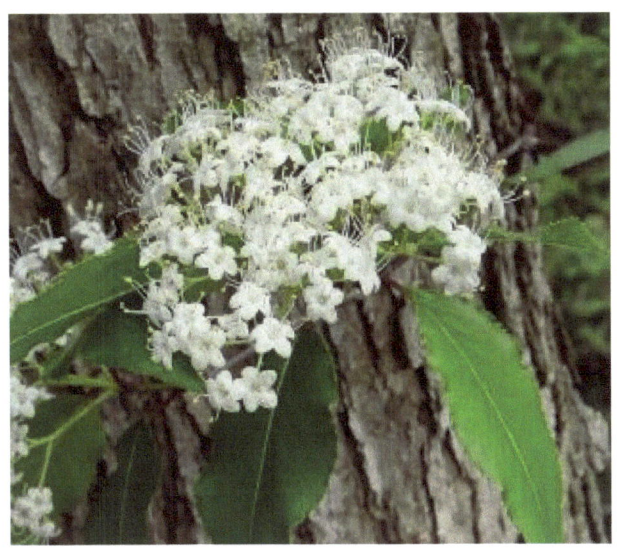

Black Haw (Bark)

Viburnum Prunifolium

Black Haw bark, sometimes known as cramp bark, has a list if things it can be used for. Women like it because it can be used to treat menstrual cramps. It is know for its effects on the uterus. It has been used by women after giving childbirth for spasms in the ureteral region. It is said to help prevent miscarriage also. A more popular use it is also known for are its effects as a sedative and muscle relaxant. The stem bark of Black Haw is approved for use in foods in the U.S.A.. It is found mostly in the eastern and southern parts of the United States. As always, the price depends on the bulk buyer in your area, but you can buy a pound of Black Haw bark for about 25.00$ a pound. So, that means you can sell it for about 25.00$ a pound to consumers.

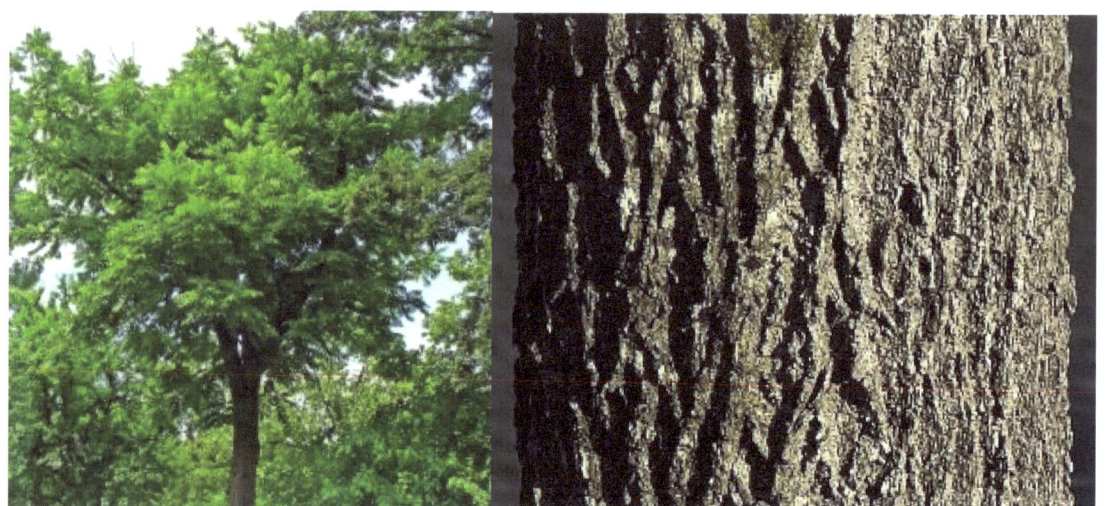

Butternut Bark

Juglans Cinerea

Butternut is a deciduous tree in the walnut family and as you can guess produces a type of nut. A deciduous tree is just a tree that loses either some or all of its leaves during a certain part of the year. Butternut tree bark is light gray in color, but can look different depending on how old the tree is. The bark typically tends to be smoother looking in the younger trees. It is sometimes known as lemon walnut or oil nut. The bark is best harvested in autumn and like most of these things, must be dried out properly before being used or sold. It can be used for constipation, gallbladder disorders, hemorrhoids, and skin diseases. In more recent years it has been used as a tonic for cancer and infections brought on by bacteria and parasites. It has properties as a laxative, analgesic, hepatic, and styptic. The price you can get for selling to a bulk buyer depends on the market as the price of all things like this fluctuates greatly, but it can be sold straight to consumers for anywhere from 20.00$ to 35.00$ a pound.

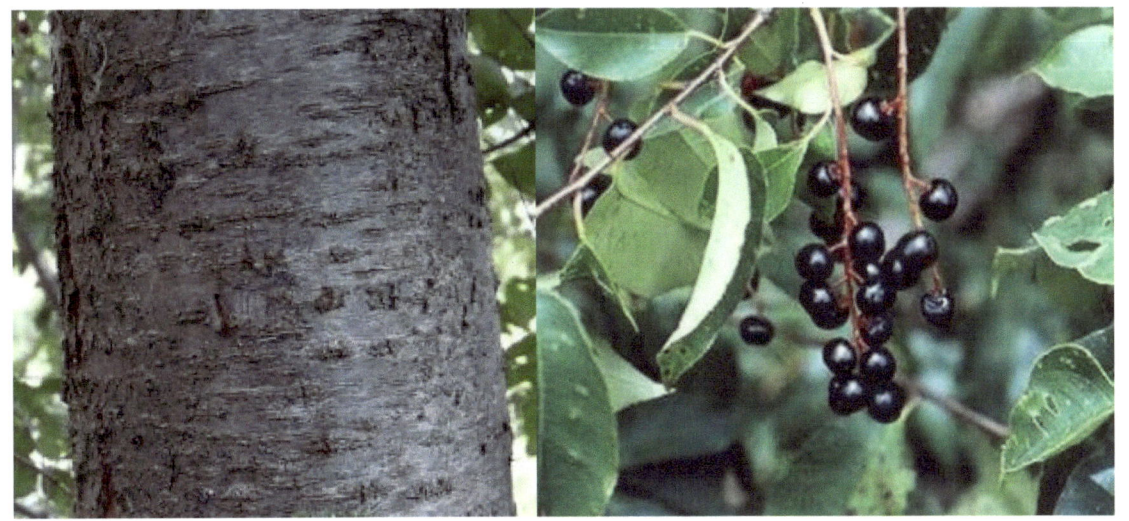

Wild Cherry Bark

Prunus Serotina

Wild Cherry, also known as black cherry because of the dark colored cherries it produces can actually be very toxic. Sometimes known as the Virginian Prune, it was used by the pioneers in the Appalachians to flavor rum or brandy. A funny thing about this tree is that is poisonous to livestock but not deer. The wilted leaves of the tree are more toxic than fresh leaves. Cherry leaves can be used to make, cyanide. Isn't that funny for such a delicious fruit. The bark can be sold in two ways. Thick bark and thin bark. Both the thick and thin bark is peeled away from the tree in a way that I described earlier. It is a brown to dark gray color and feels very rough or ribbed. The thin bark is usually smooth with a light gray color. The leaves are the most toxic part of this tree and while I would not try this myself the bark is used in cough syrups because of its sedative, expectorant, drying, and cough-suppressing effects. It is used to make medicine for colds, whooping cough, bronchitis and other lung problems. It is also used for diarrhea, gout, digestive disorders, pain, and cancer. While being used for many things, you should really know what you are doing before attempting anything with this. People that do things like this have acquired the knowledge over a lifetime of experience. I have personally seen the leaves be made into a poison to keep things like rodents out of the house and pests out of the garden. That is the way they used to do it. This is one of those things you should be really careful with. The leaves and bark are safe to handle, just do not ingest any of the leaves. The price you can get for a pound of black cherry bark depends on the bulk buyer in your area, but there is a demand for it. It is sold to consumers for around 6.00$ to 9.00$ a pound. You would probably be surprised how many things around you can kill you and how many plants can be used to make poison. Maybe I will write something about that in the future.

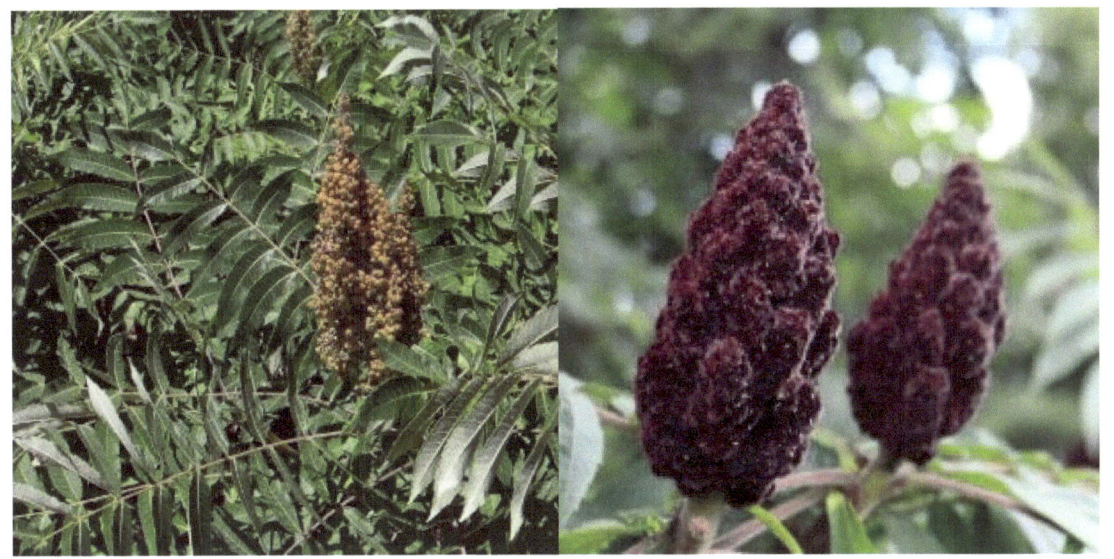

Sumac Tree (Bark)

Rhus Glabra

Not to be confused with poison sumac (Toxicodendron Vernix), the smooth sumac tree does not cause itchy rashes. The two do look similar but poison sumac is generally a small tree that grows in low wetland areas and have grayish white berries that hang down from the tree. Vine and shrub-like poison ivy and oak have three distinct leaflets per leaf, making them stand out and easy to recognize. Sometimes known as fragrant sumac or aromatic sumac, some actually use this tree for landscaping or in their garden. The name sumac comes from an old Syrian word meaning (red), because in the autumn the leaves will turn a reddish to purple color. Only the female plants grow the berry clusters. In the old days Native Americans and colonists used the sumac to make pipe stems for their pipes because the trunks are known to be hollow. While the berries are high in vitamin C and can be made into something like lemonade, there is a demand for the bark and roots of this tree. The roots are harvested in the fall of the year and must be dried before being sold. Parts of smooth sumac were valued by Native American tribes for a whole list of uses. (Sore throat treatment, ear medicine, eye medicine, astringent, heart medicine, venereal aid, ulcer treatment, treatment for rashes, antiemetic, antidiarrheal, antihemorrhagic, blister treatment, cold remedy, emetic, mouthwash, asthma treatment, tuberculosis remedy) Parts of the tree were also used by Native Americans to create dye. There are many different ways you can use this tree and make money from its parts. The price per pound of its bark and roots varies depending on demand and region.

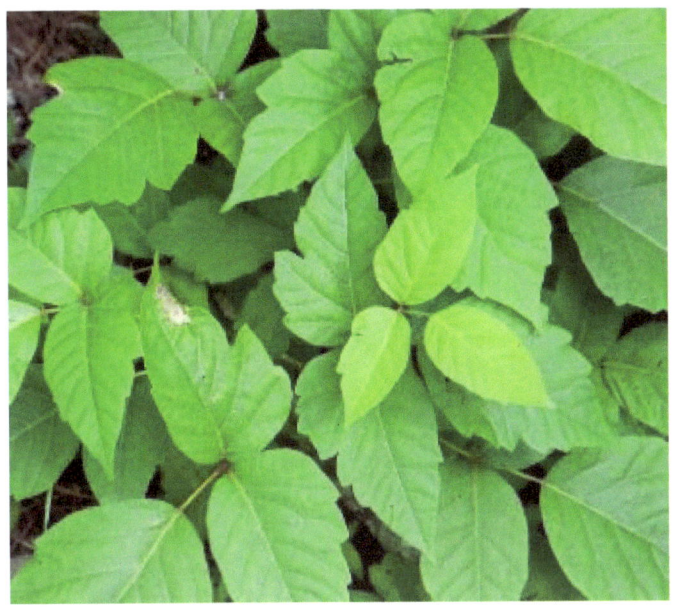

Poison Ivy

Toxicodendron Radicans

I would normally not even talk about this, but since we just covered Smooth Sumac which is related to poison sumac, I want to include poison ivy. First, it may surprise you to find out that you can actually sell poison ivy leaf. The reason I felt it important to include this is so you, the reader, can identify it when out hunting. Notice how the leaves grow in sections of three. This is what to look for when out in the wild. When you see a vine or a bush that has leaves like this and you do not know what it is, then it is best to stay away from it. I myself am not allergic to it, but some can just walk by this plant and find themselves in the hospital. Besides wanting to include it for identification purposes, it will surprise you to learn that poison ivy leaf can be harvested, dried, and sold for around 2.00$ a pound but like with all of this stuff, the price fluctuates. It is best to contact your local bulk buyer and ask what their prices and needs are. The plant can be used to treat pain, rheumatoid arthritis, menstrual period problems, swelling, and itchy skin disorders.

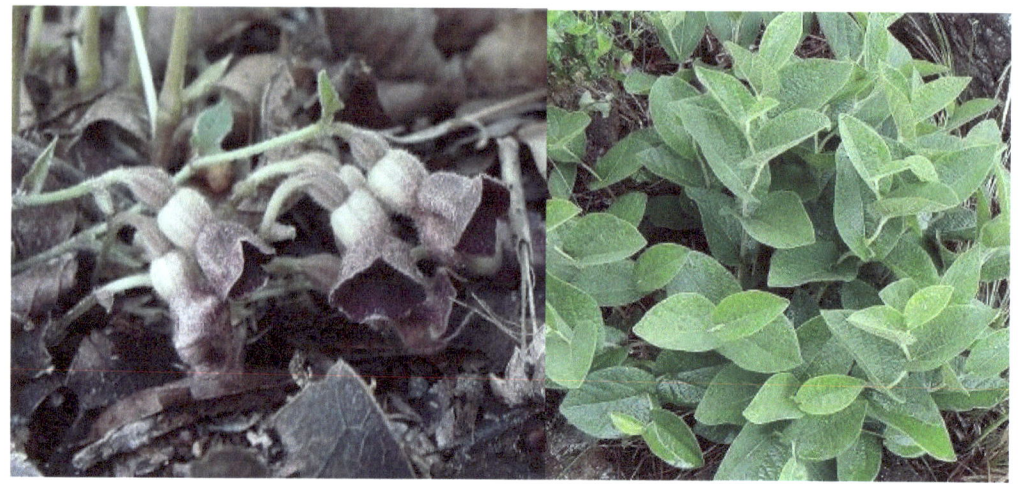

Virginia and Texas Snakeroot

Aristolochia Reticulata

Texas snake root (shown above) is also known as Texas Dutchman's Pipe. There are a few different varieties of plants with the name "snakeroot" attached to it and they are all very different plants. Depending on where you live the names may change. The snakeroot I was used to digging had a very unique smell to it. These are non-woody woodland perennials of the Aristolochiaceae (Birthwort) Family. Texas Dutchman's-pipe and Virginia snakeweed are important host plants for pipevine swallowtail butterflies. By eating the aristolochic acids in the plants, caterpillars and butterflies take on a bad taste keeping them safe from most predators. These plants are known to grow in well-drained, rocky or sandy woodlands and like partially shady to mostly sunny areas.

Continued on next page-

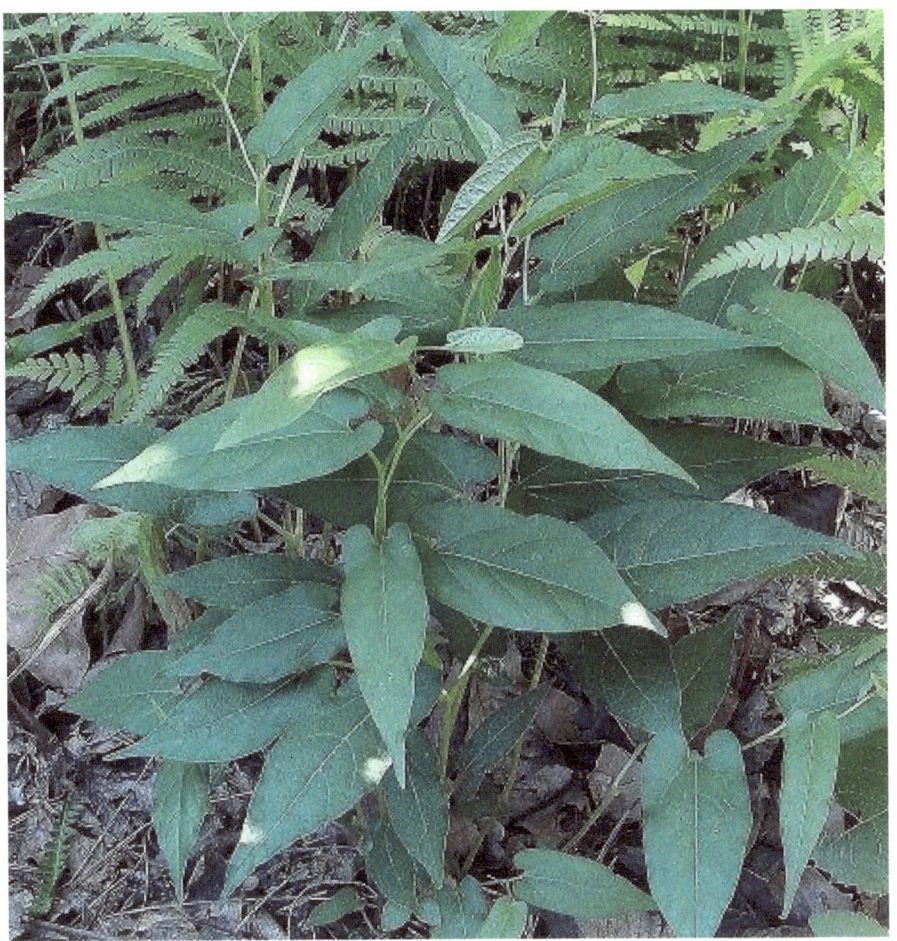

Virginia Snakeroot

Aristolochia Serpentari

Virginia snakeroot gets its name because it was once used to treat snakebites. While these two plants grow really similar flowers the stems of Virginia snakeroot are thinner and weaker than Texas Dutchman's-pipe and may recline on the ground. This is one of the plants that has a lot of value. While prices fluctuate, a pound of Texas and Virginia snake root is worth generally around a 100.00$ a pound.

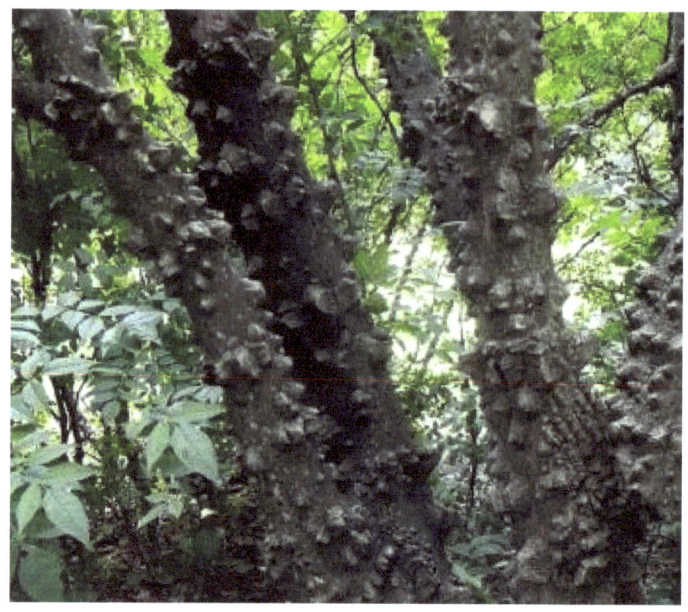

(Southern) Prickly Ash Bark

Zanthoxylum Clava-Herculis

Called the southern prickly ash because it is native to the south eastern United States and the bark is...prickly. The bark and berries from this tree can be used to make medicine. Some of the medicines that can be made from this tree are used to treat poor circulation in the legs and fingers, menstrual cramps, joint pain, toothaches, sores, and ulcers. Some use this tree to make a tonic that they use as a stimulant and is sometimes used to break a fever by causing sweating. A bit of interesting information is that southern prickly ash is one of the ingredients in "Hoxsey cure" for cancer. Once dried properly a pound of prickly ash bark will fetch you around 3.00$ a pound. As always, the price fluctuates due to region and demand.

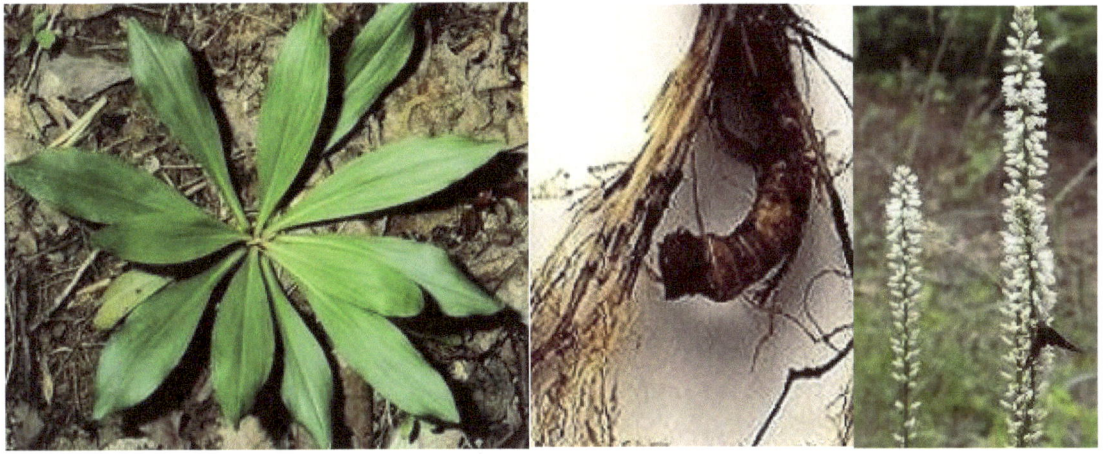

Star Grub Root

Chamaelirium Luteum

Star grub root, sometimes known as false unicorn was used by Native Americans mainly for women to relieve menstrual cramps. Also believed to improve fertility and prevent miscarriage, is known to have anti-inflammatory effects. Harvesting of the roots usually occurs in autumn, after flowering is complete, and when plants are about four to eight years old. The main bioactive components of star root are a mixture of steroidal saponins, including chamaelirin and aglycone diosgenin that can cause vomiting and menstrual discharge. This root is a one of the more valuable ones you can find. While the price will wildly fluctuate, a pound of this root can fetch you anywhere between 50.00$ a pound to 200.00$ a pound. Contact your local bulk buyer to see what kind of prices they have.

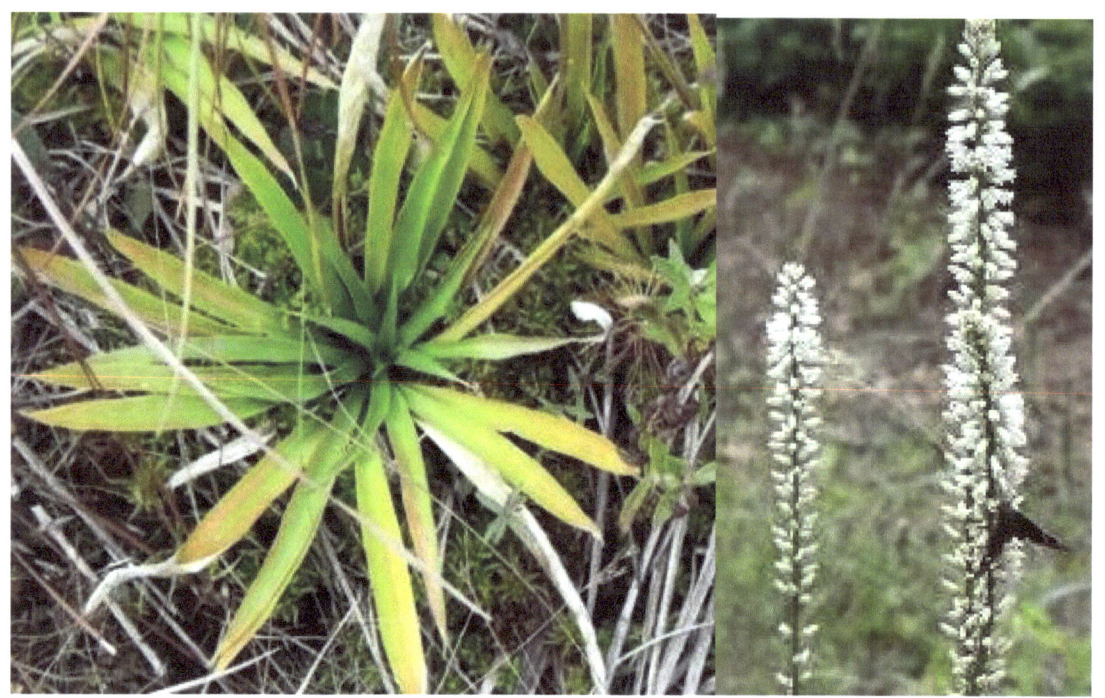

Star Grass Root

Aletris Farinosa

Star grass root (not to be confused for star grub root or false unicorn) is also sometimes knows as True Unicorn. Also, not to be confused with Giant Star Grass (Cynodon Plectostachyus). True unicorn is harvested commercially in Virginia, Tennessee, and North Carolina. It is known to have a sweet taste becoming bitter and soapy. Caution, use only under professional guidance. Once again, I remind you that people who do this have acquired knowledge over a lifetime of experience. The dried rhizome (part of the root) can be toxic if overdosed, causing colic, diarrhea, and vomiting but is safe to handle. Star grass is a perennial native to eastern North America. While price fluctuates you can expect somewhere around 20.00$ for a pound of this root.

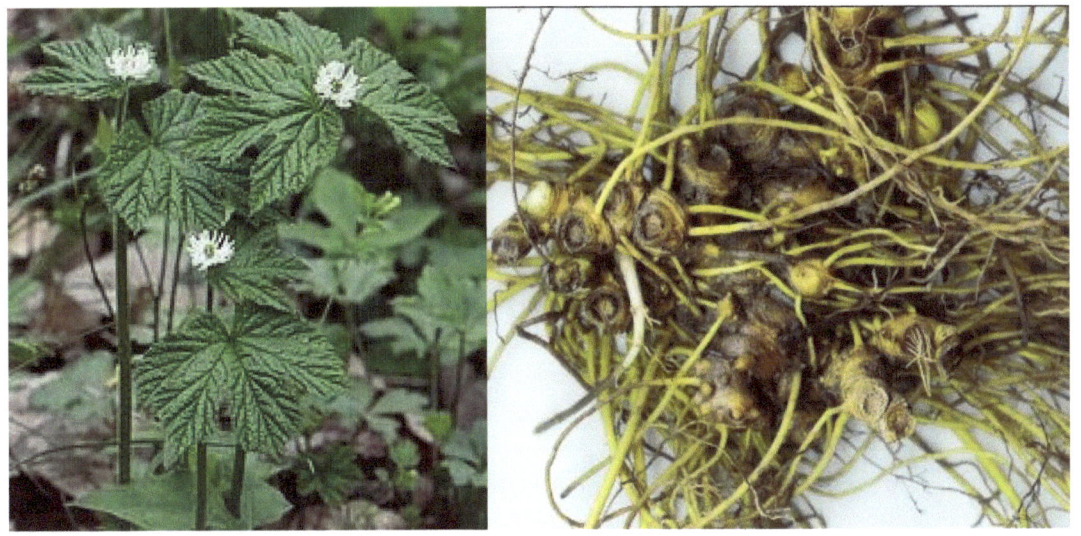

Golden Seal Root

Hydrastis Canadensis

Golden Seal is related to the May Apple plant. Both the herb and root from this plant can be sold. This can be found for sale almost everywhere in stores. It is widely rumored that Golden Seal will help you pass a drug test. When I was much younger a military recruiter told some of us to take it before we went in for drug screening during recruitment. There is no proof that it actually works for this, but it is famous for it. It does have a large list of other things it can be used for. Urinary tract infections, vaginal pain, menstrual period problems, skin rashes, itching, eczema, herpes blisters, cold sores, mouthwash for sore gums and mouth, acne, dandruff, ringworm, liver disorders, cancer, chronic fatigue syndrome, anorexia, jaundice, gonorrhea, fever, pneumonia, malaria, ears for ringing, earache, and deafness. The list goes on. You can expect somewhere around 4.00$ a pound for the herb and around 22.00$ a pound for the root.

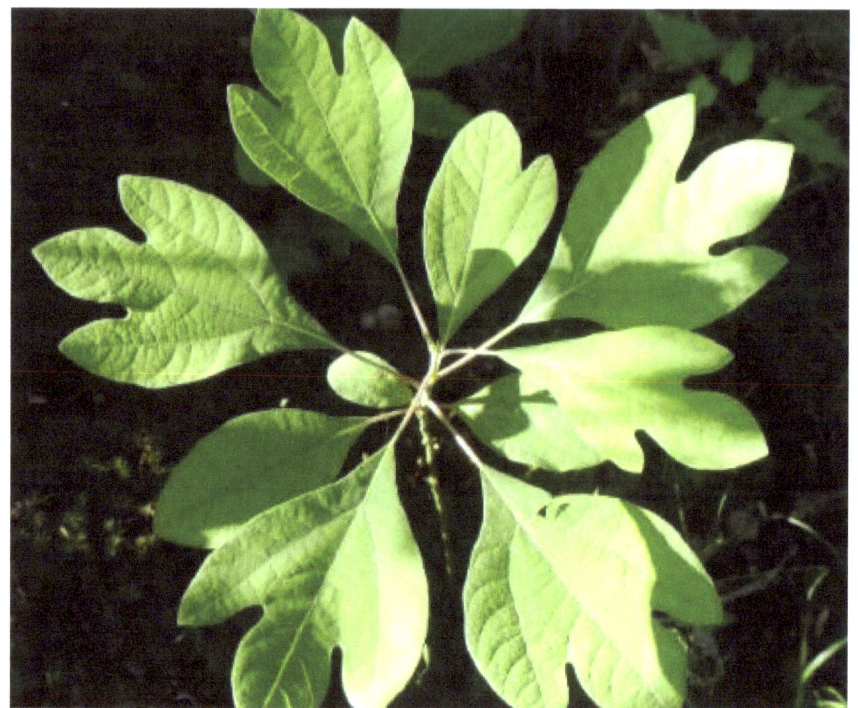

Sassafras Leaf

Scientific Name = Sassafras

Sassafras is a pretty common plant native to eastern North America and East Asia. It is the primary ingredient in traditional root beer and can also be used to make a drug known as MDMA. There are lots of controversies and conspiracy theories relating to Sassafras and its active compound, safrole. Safrole is a volatile oil that the FDA banned as a potential carcinogen in the 1960s. Sassafras Leaf can still be legally sold as a topical skin wash or as aromatic potpourri. I find this a very interesting plant. You can get about a 1.00$ a pound for the leaf of the plant with no stem. When you sell the things, you harvest they must be prepared correctly and dried properly of the buyer will "dock" you.

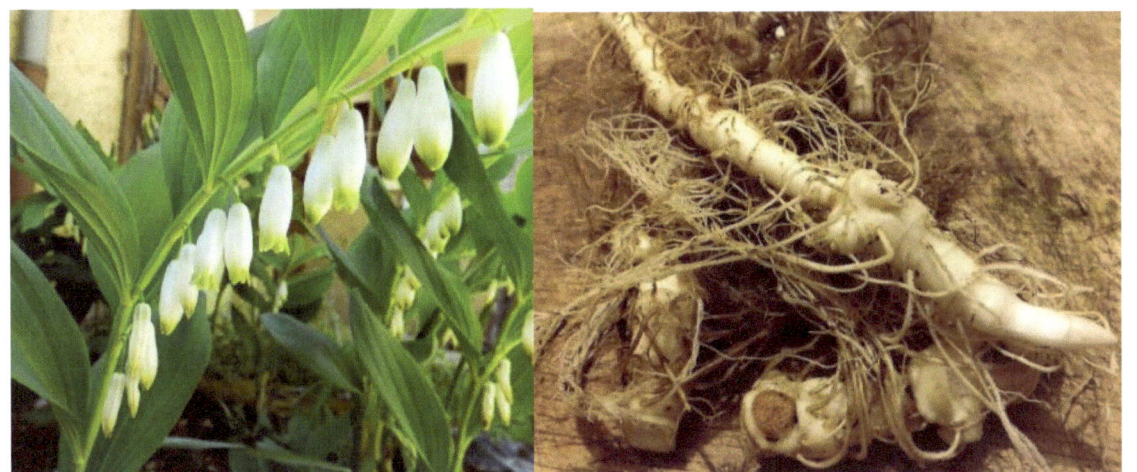

Solomon Seal Root

Polygonatum Biflorum

Solomon Seal is quite common in Appalachia. It is commonly used to treat lung disorders, inflammation, and to dry out tissue and draw it together (that is an astringent). Some people apply Solomon's seal directly to the skin for bruises, ulcers, or boils on the fingers, hemorrhoids, skin redness, and water retention. Those are some of the many uses for this root. While not worth as much as some of the other things you can harvest, it makes up for this in how common it is. You can expect a respectable 4.00$ a pound for this root.

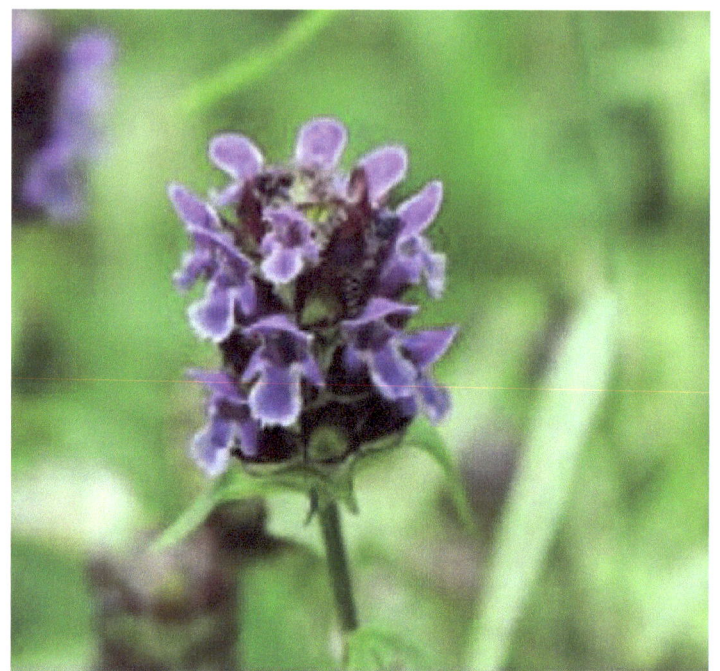

Heal All

Prunella Vulgaris

An interesting name, Prunella Vulgaris, you can guess by the name (heal all) what the plant is used for. Heal-all is a perennial herb found throughout Europe, Asia and North America. For maximum potency heal all herb should be harvested during the mature flowering stage from June to September. All parts above the ground can be harvested. The herb is used for mouth and throat ulcers, sore throat, and internal bleeding. Some people are known to use heal-all for HIV/AIDS, fever, headache, dizziness, liver disease, and muscle spasm. It is also used to kill germs (as an antiseptic), loosen phlegm (as an expectorant), and tighten and dry skin (as an astringent). Some have been said to use this plant to treat herpes. It is a good little plant all the way around and very common. While prices fluctuate due to demand and region, you can expect around 0.50$ a pound for the Heal-All herb.

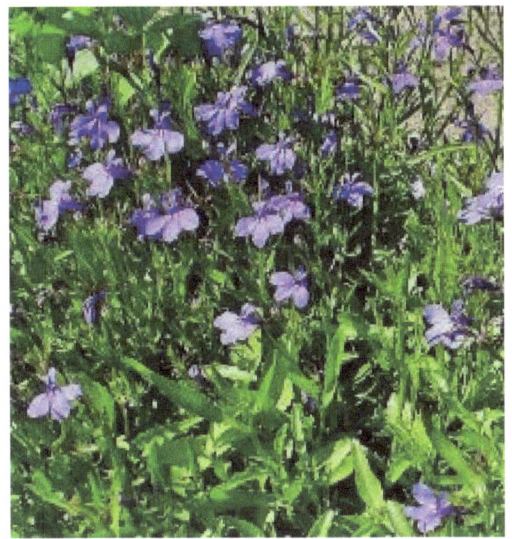

Lobelia Herb

Lobelia inflata

Lobelia herb is also known as "Indian Tobacco". It is called this because Native Americans were known to smoke this as a treatment for asthma. The parts of the plant that are above ground can be used to make a few different medicines. While some are said to use this plant as a way to relax, others use it to treat breathing problems such as asthma, bronchitis, whooping cough, and shortness of breath in newborn infants. Shortness of breath while you sleep is known as apnea. Lobelia is a stimulant and may raise your blood pressure. I must state again, if making your own home remedies, do so with great care. You do this at your own risk. While you are not likely to encounter any problems, there are other side effects to these plants and herbs. Lobelia may cause other problems if taken incorrectly in large amounts. Lobelia Herb is native to eastern North America and can be found quite commonly. You can expect to gain around 3.00$ a pound from a bulk buyer.

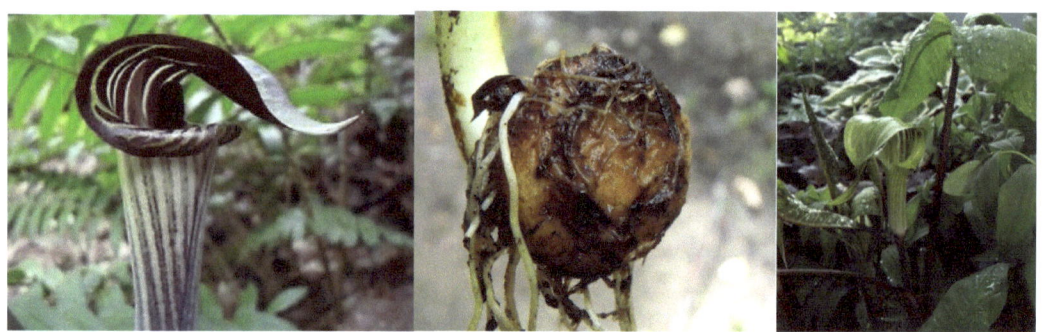

Indian Turnip root

Arisaema Triphyllum

The Indian Turnip root is also called "Jack in the Pulpit". It has another host of names that it is also known by depending on where you live or which variety of the plant you find. Such as bog onion, brown dragon, dragon-root, wake-robin, or wild turnip. It was commonly used by Native Americans for stomach and bowel problems. It grows in the wild regions of mainly the eastern part of North America but can be cultivated anywhere. It is known to grow by streams and places that are really moist. The root is harvested in the fall and tubers (stems from the root) may need to be sliced to aid in the drying. In the later 19th century, the Indian Turnip was used in medicines for a variety of things. Such as cough, colds, snakebites, asthma, rheumatism, lockjaw, swelling of the hands and feet, facial paralysis, numbness, dizziness, strokes, flatulence, hoarseness, stomatitis, and spasms. Sometimes it would be made into a poultice for things like boils, sores, ulcers, ringworm, abscesses, and a gargle for the mouth. Some Native Americans would dry and powder the plant as a cure for headache while other used it (believe it or not) as a form of birth control or temporary sterility. You can expect around a 1.00$ a pound to a bulk root buyer, though prices fluctuate.

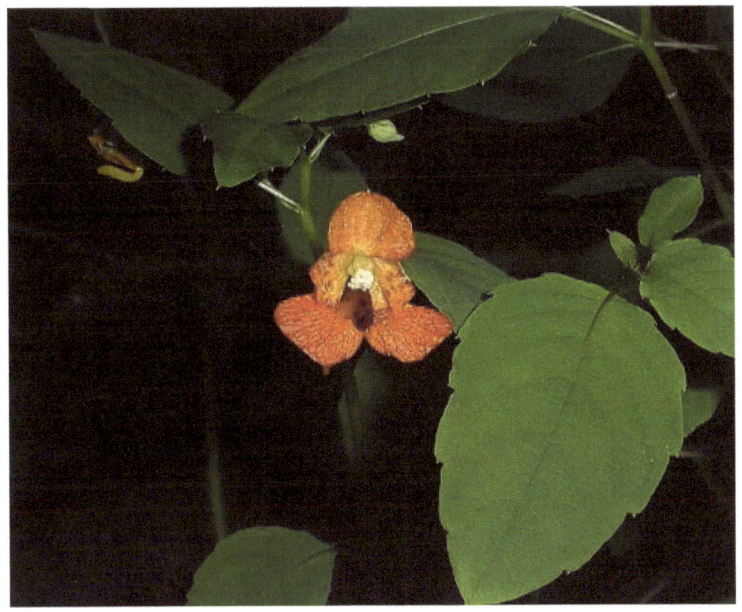

Jewel weed

Impatiens Capensis

Jewel Weed or Orange Jewel Weed is also called the "Spotted Touch Me Not" because of the red spots that form on the orange flower. The plant flowers June through September. Fruits grow in long green pods that pop when touched, dispersing the seeds. It is known to grow in dense thicketed areas that are moist and shady. It is commonly found along streams. The leaves can be crushed and formed into a poultice that is used to cure poison ivy. One thing about nature is that usually when you have something that can harm you growing in an area (such as Poison Ivy), the cure will often also be growing around or close to the same area (such as Jewel Weed). The poison and the antidote often grow beside each other, and there are lots of poisons in nature. Tea made from the leaves is said to prevent breaking out from Poison Ivy. Jewelweed contains a compound called "lawsone" in its leaves proven to have anti-histamine and anti-inflammatory properties. It grows all over North America and you can expect to gain around 0.50$ a pound.

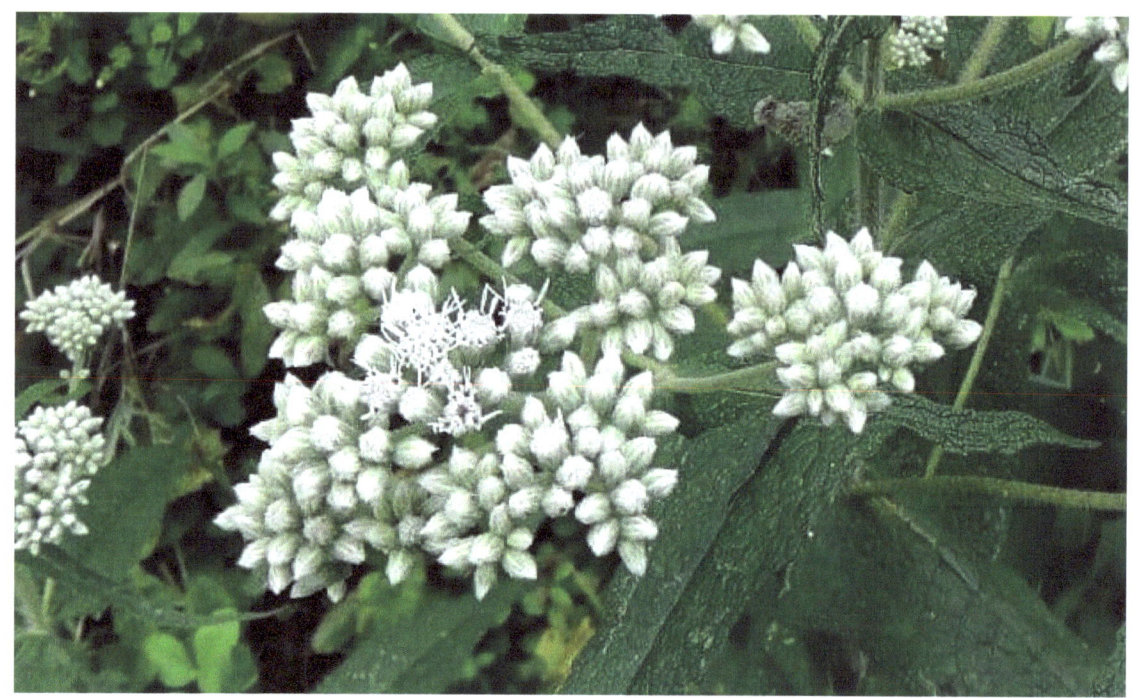

Boneset Herb

Eupatorium Perfoliatum

Boneset Herb also called agueweed, feverwort, or sweating-plant is a North American perennial plant in the Aster family. Native Americans used Boneset Herb as a remedy, for antipyretic (to reduce fever). The early settlers in North America used the plant to treat a variety of things. Such as rheumatism (joint pain), dropsy, dengue fever, malaria, pneumonia, and influenza. It can also be used to treat acute bronchitis, nasal inflammation, fluid retention, pneumonia, and as a stimulant to cause sweating. Some other things Boneset can be used for is to increase urine output, cause vomiting, and treat constipation. Boneset contains chemicals that might work like anti-cancer medications. It also might have some mild anti-bacterial properties. Liking to grow in moist places, you can get around 0.50$ a pound for this herb.

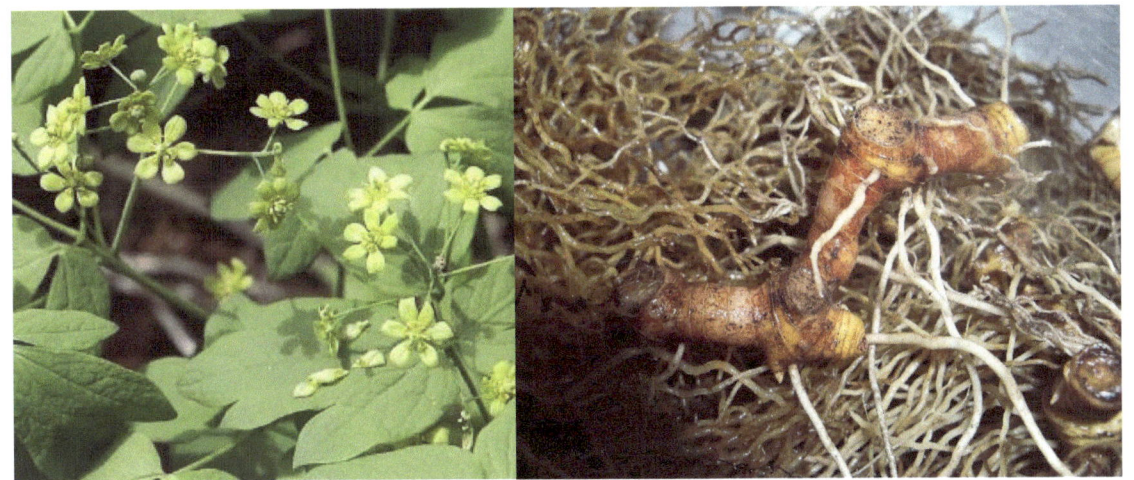

Blue Cohosh Root

Caulophyllum Thalictroides

Blue cohosh, also called squaw root or papoose root, is a flowering plant in the Berberidaceae family. It will grow blue berry-like fruits. Believe it or not, this herb can be used to induce labor, but mainly it is the root which is sought out for sale. Still, some of the things this flower can be used for are stimulating the uterus and starting labor, starting menstruation, stopping muscle spasms, a laxative, treating colic, sore throat, cramps, hiccups, epilepsy, hysterics, inflammation of the uterus, infection of the female organs (pelvic inflammatory disease), over-growth of uterine tissue (endometriosis), and joint conditions. "Cohosh" is from the Algonquin Indian word meaning "rough". Blue Cohosh is native to the moist woodlands of the upper Appalachian Mountain Range. You can get around a 1.50$ a pound for the root to bulk buyers. Remember the roots must be cleaned and properly dried.

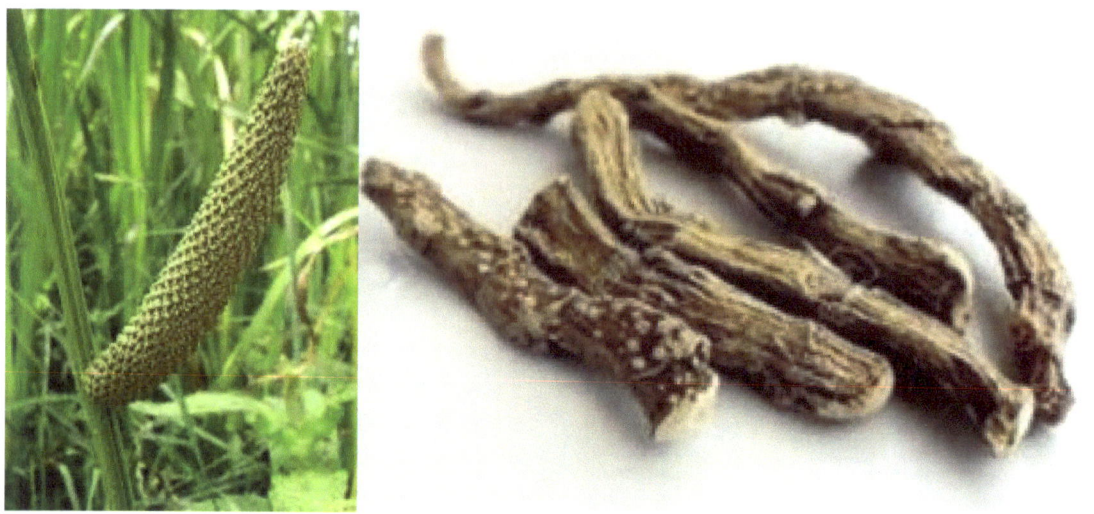

Calamus Root

Acorus Calamus

Calamus Root is also sometimes known as "Sweet Flag". It is a perennial semi-aquatic plant that likes to grow in marshes and on the muddy banks of streams. This plant was used by Native Americans to attract muskrats, which were valued for their furs. Calamus is commonly used in bath additives, gargles, lotions, or washes. Though not recommended for internal use by the FDA and despite safety concerns, the root can be mixed and used in combination with other things to create medicines for different stomach problems, including ulcers, inflammation of the stomach lining (gastritis), diarrhea, intestinal gas (flatulence), upset stomach, and many more. Calamus is mentioned or referenced in the bible in Exodus 3: 2325, Isaiah 43: 24, Jeremiah 6:2, and Ezekiel 27:19. Song of Solomon 4:14 indicates that "calamus" was grown as a garden plant. Acorus calamus is a plant that grows in wet areas. You can get around 3.50$ a pound for the root of this plant to bulk buyers.

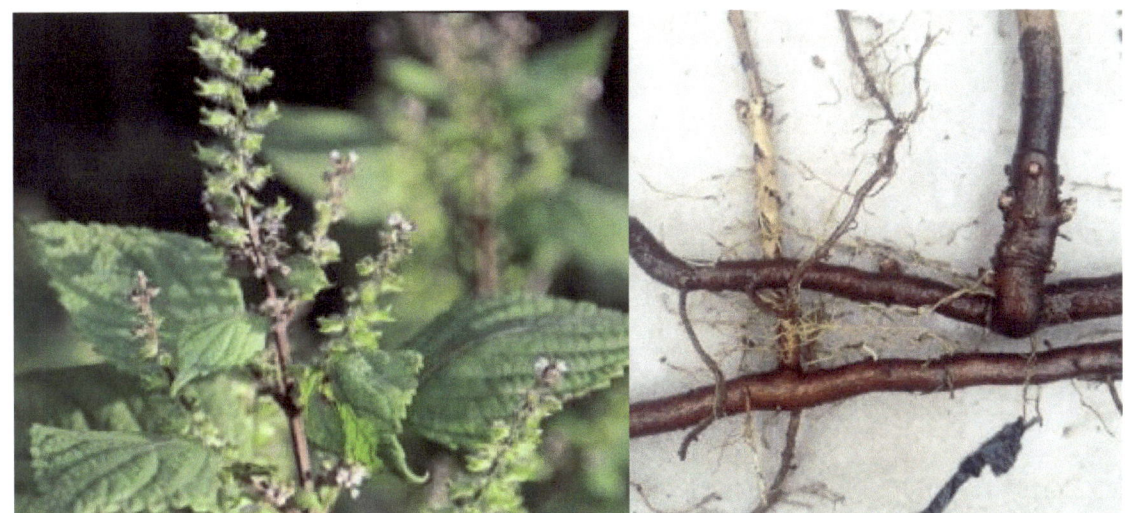

Black Indian Hemp Root

Apocynum Cannabinum

Black Indian Hemp Root is also sometimes called dogbane, Amy root, hemp dogbane, prairie dogbane, Indian hemp, rheumatism root, or wild cot ton. It is a perennial herbaceous plant that grows throughout much of North America and is poisonous. Apocynum means "poisonous to dogs". Although poisonous, the roots are used for heart stimulants. The leaves can be mashed and used to make remedies for rheumatism and applied to wounds. Some Native Americans would make charms with the plant to be used against 'bad medicine' or evil influence. While I remind you to use care if using this root, the same is true for all medicines. All medicines are poison. This plant is not poisonous to humans (or at least no cases have ever been reported), but it can be to your pets and livestock. This plant has also been used for coughs, pox, whooping cough, asthma, internal parasites, diarrhea and also to increase milk flow in lactating mothers. You can expect around 4.00$ a pound for the root of this plant to bulk buyers.

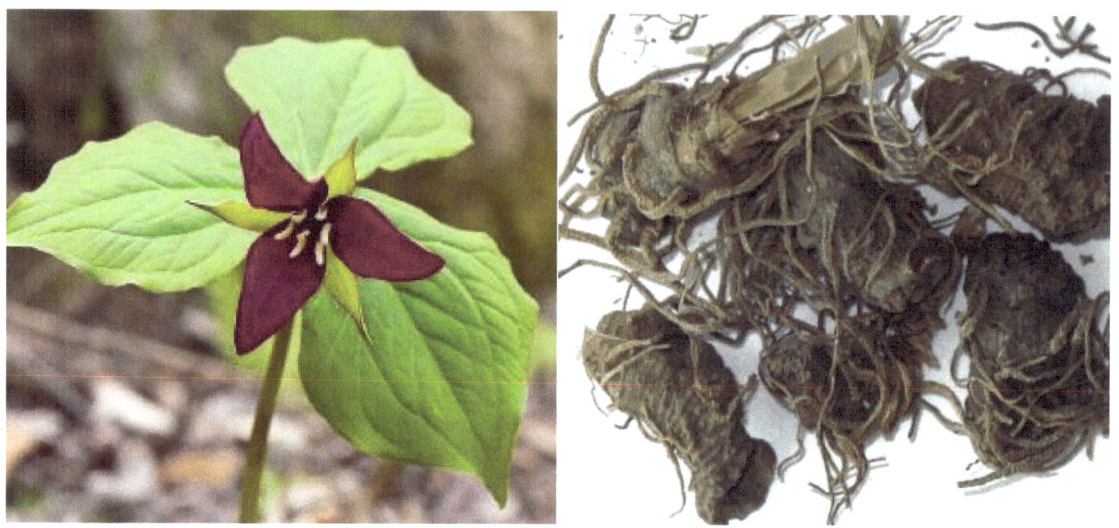

Beth Root

Trillium Erectum

Beth Root is also sometimes known as red trillium, wake-robin, purple trillium, stinking Benjamin, and many more. The root, underground stem (rhizome), and leaf are used to make medicine. Despite safety concerns, some women take Beth root for heavy and painful menstrual periods. Beth root is also used for reducing swelling and for breaking up chest congestion. Some people make a poultice and apply Beth root directly to the skin for varicose veins, ulcers, bruises, and bleeding hemorrhoids. It is also used orally as an astringent and expectorant. Beth root is unsafe to consume orally because it is a known gastrointestinal irritant. Ingesting large amounts of Beth root in plant or oil form may cause vomiting. Bulk root buyers will pay around 2.00$ a pound for this root cleaned and dried.

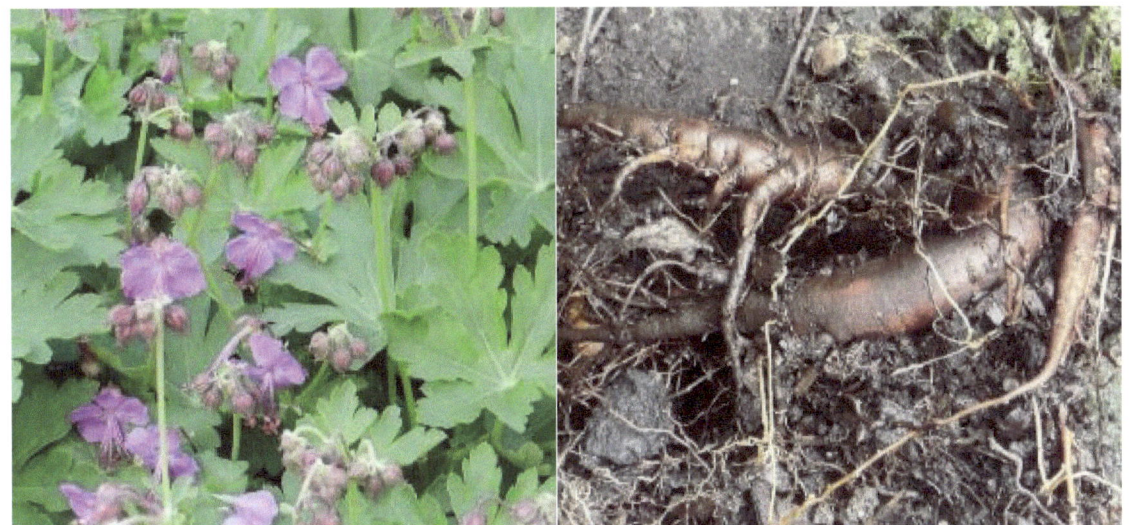

Cranesbill Root

Geranium Maculatum

Cranesbill Root is also sometimes known as alumroot, storks-bill, and wild geranium. The American cranesbill is one of the many plants of the Geranium family that is used in herbal medicine. Sometimes used to make an eyewash, the powdered root, often mixed with other herbs, was used as a compress on wounds and swollen feet. Teas and tinctures can also be made from parts of this plant. Cranesbill is indigenous to the eastern and central North America. It is mostly found growing wild in woods and forests. Cranesbill is used for the tannins it produces, compounds that cause proteins in mucous membranes and other linings of the human body exposed directly to the tea to cross-link. The Cranesbill Root, must be harvested in late February or March before the signature purple flowers appear, since this is when the tannic acid in Cranesbill Root is at its most potent levels. You can expect around 3.50$ for a pound of this root.

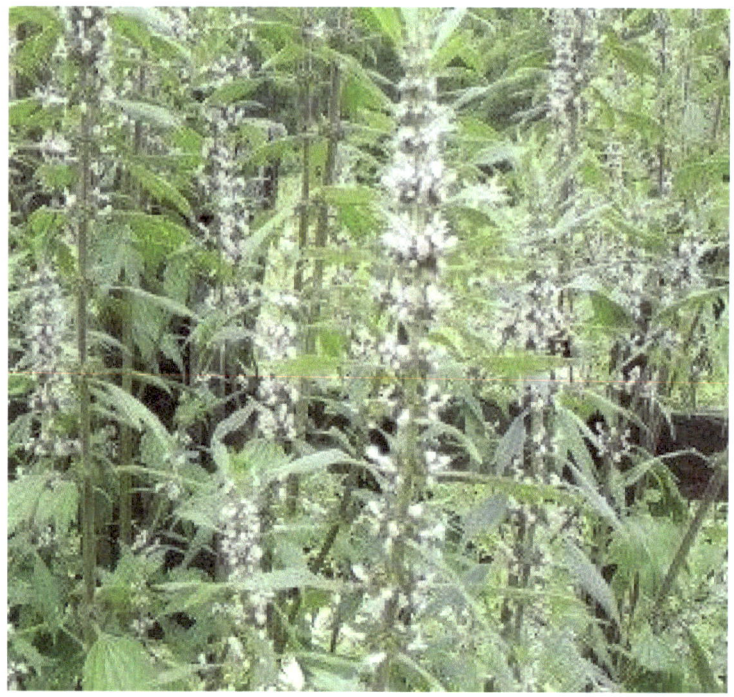

Mothers-wort Herb

Leonurus Cardiaca

Other common names for Mothers-wort include throw-wort, lion's ear, and lion's tail. The parts that grow above the ground (the herb) are used to make medicine. Motherwort is used for heart conditions, including heart failure, irregular heartbeat, and heart symptoms due to anxiety. Some people apply motherwort directly to the skin for wounds, itching and shingles. It has many more uses, mostly for women and some uses for cancer.

Mothers-wort may trigger a number of side effects, such as diarrhea, drowsiness, sedation, altered heart rate and rhythm, low blood pressure, and uterine bleeding and contractions. Pregnant women and people with low blood pressure should avoid using this herb.

Mothers-wort grows well in waste places that are moist and often on gravelly or calcareous soils. It can grow in sunny or lightly shaded areas. You can expect around 0.50$ a pound.

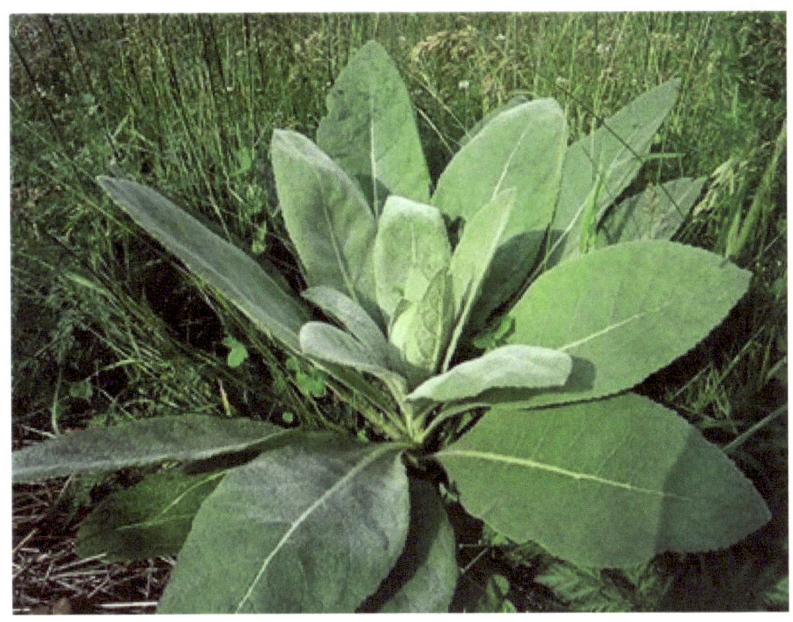

Mullein Herb and Leaf

Verbascum Densiflorum

Mullein is sometimes also known as Aaron's rod. Common mullein or Great Mullein, is a species of mullein native to Europe, northern Africa, and Asia, that was introduced in the Americas. Mullein is a biennial herbaceous member of the Scrophulariaceae family. It has been used historically for lung conditions. Ashes from the leaf were used to darken the hair and the yellow leaves were used to lighten it. The leaves were dried, rolled and used as wicks for candles and the entire dried flowering stalks were dipped in tallow and used for torches, hence the names 'candlewick plant' or 'torches'. This plant has a long and interesting history. Some people take mullein by mouth for breathing conditions such as cough or asthma, pneumonia, colds, and sore throat. You can expect around 0.50$ a pound for this herb from bulk buyers.

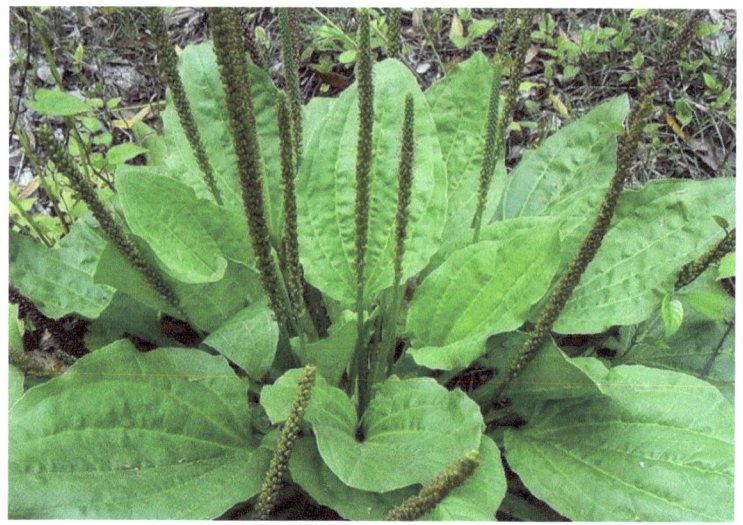

Plantain Leaf

Plantago Major

Plantain leaf is a common backyard herb. Native Americans used plantain leaves to relieve the pain of bee stings and insect bites, stop the itching of poison ivy and other allergic rashes, and promote healing in sores and bruises. Plantain tea can be used as a mouthwash to help heal and prevent sores in the mouth, and as an expectorant. It is said that Plantain can help heal the damaged gut or urinary system. It may be used best as a dried herb in tea or in a tincture as a remedy for 'wounds on the inside. This plant is a wild edible that is good for overall health and it can be used to treat chronic diarrhea as well as digestive tract disorders. Broadleaf plantain is packed with nutrients and is safe to ingest. Some side effects such as diarrhea may be associated with this plant and some may have allergic reactions. So, as always, use care. It is a very common plant and you can expect around 0.50 a pound for the dried leaves of this plant.

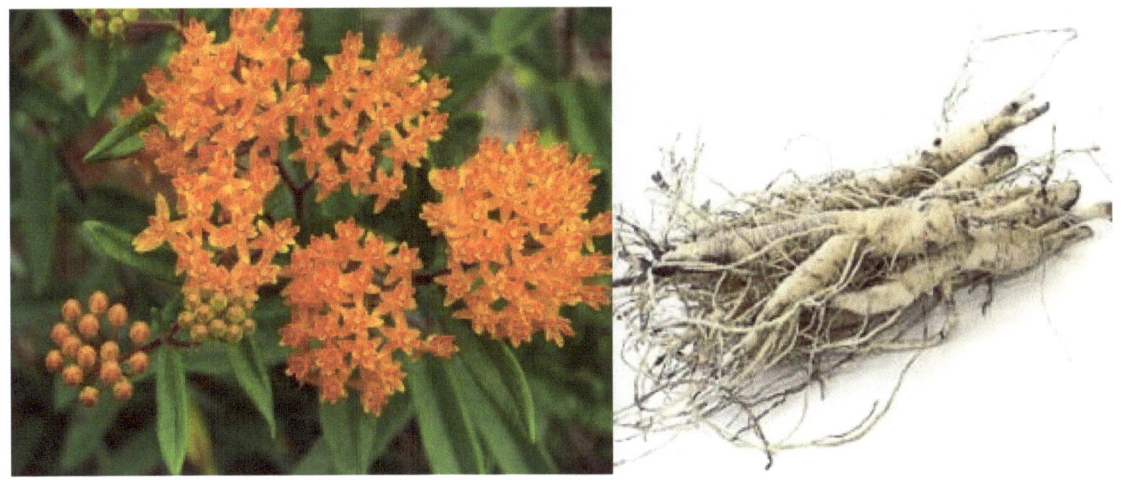

Pleurisy Root

Asclepias Tuberosa

Pleurisy Root, or "Orange butterfly weed" is a species of milkweed native to eastern North America. It is commonly known as butterfly weed because of the butterflies that are attracted to the plant by its color and the production of its nectar. It is also the larval food plant of the queen and monarch butterflies. The root is used as medicine. Pleurisy is a swelling of the lining of the lungs, which is where the name comes from since this plant is used to treat this condition. Despite serious safety concerns, pleurisy root is used for coughs, swelling of the air sacs in the lungs, swelling of the airways (bronchitis), and influenza. This herb grows primarily in the southwestern and midwestern United States. For maximum potency Pleurisy root should be harvested in the late summer or fall after the growth has stopped and the seed pods have appeared. This plant may also be used to treat disorders of the uterus, muscle spasms, and pain. It is thought to loosen mucus so it can be coughed up as well to promote sweating. You can gain a modest 4.00$ a pound for this root after it has been cleaned and dried.

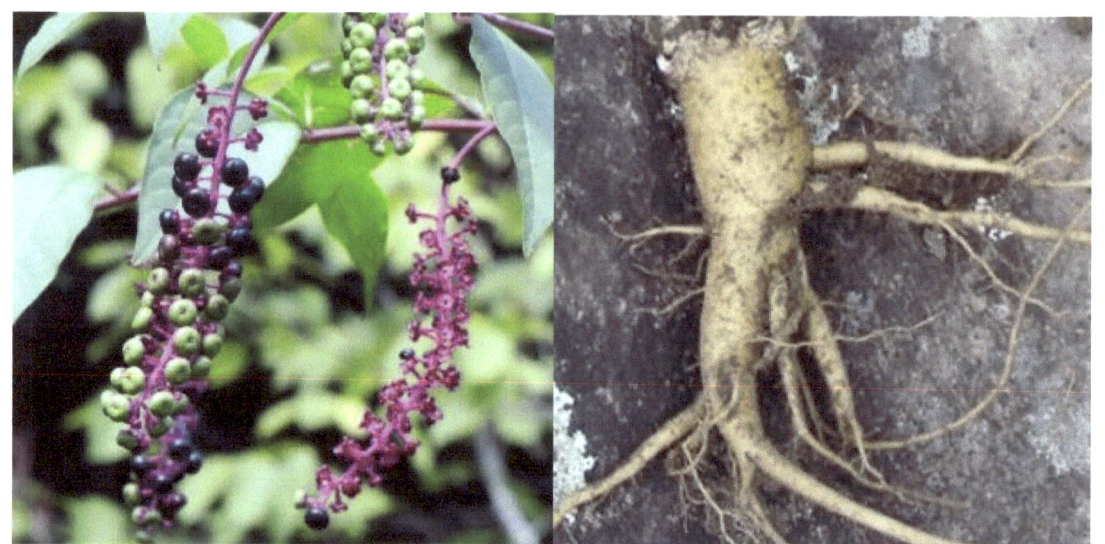

Poke Root

Phytolacca

Poke Root is a perennial plant native to North America. WARNING: All parts of the pokeweed plant, especially the root, are poisonous. Do not touch pokeweed with your bare hands. Chemicals in the plant can pass through the skin and affect the blood. Before using the leaves, herbalists have to boil them three times, discarding the water in-between to create a dish that is referred to as "poke salad" or "polk salad. The "polk salad" we gather in my area is a completely different plant. It is basically wild lettuce. Remember, depending on where you live, some of these plants may go by different names. Sometimes known as nightshade, the berries were once used to create and ink and dye. Elvis wrote a song about this plant called, "Polk Salad Annie". Native Americans used this plant for a myriad of conditions including as a heart stimulant, for rheumatism, arthritis, dysentery, and cancer. Always use caution when collecting and harvesting wild herbs, roots, plants, and barks. You can expect around 0.50$ a pound for this root after it is cleaned and dried.

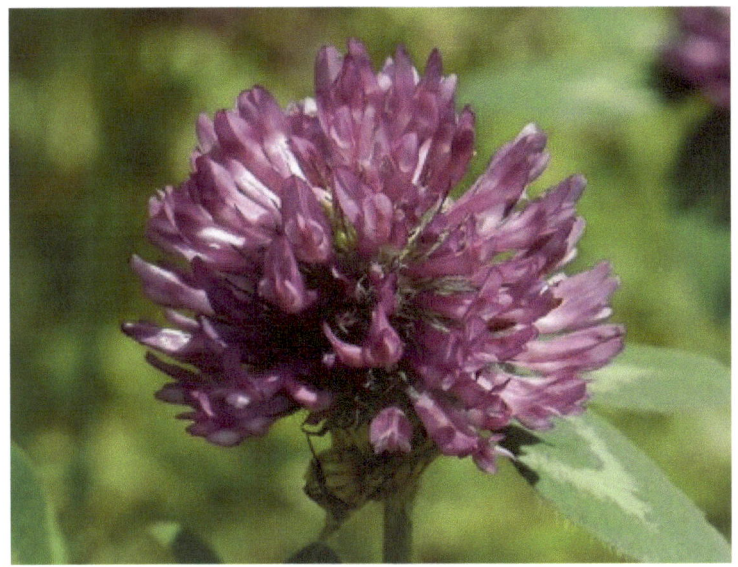

Red Clover Blossom

Trifolium Pratense

Red Clover Blossom is an herbaceous species of flowering plant, a low growing perennial. These are very common and you may see them everywhere, but it may surprise you to learn that it is not native to North America. Originally this plant was found in northwest Africa, Asia, and Europe, but it has been cultivated and naturalized in many parts of the world. The flowers are collected in full bloom, during the summer months and dried. This flower has some religious significance in history amongst Druids and Medieval Christians. Some of the uses of this flower include helping children with persistent cough, raising good cholesterol, and preventing blood clots and promoting blood flow. Some studies show it may slow the growth of some cancers, but due to its estrogen like qualities, it may not be good for breast cancer. It is also a wild edible that is high in many nutrients and vitamins. While being a common flower, you can make a respectable 3.50$ a pound for the dried-out herb from bulk buyers. Maybe more if sold direct to the consumer.

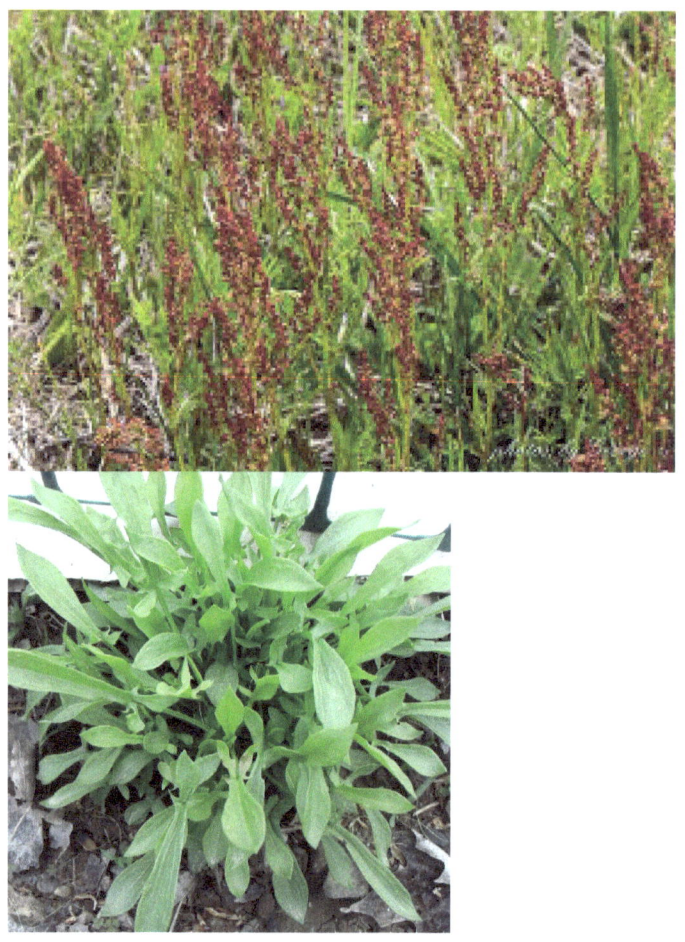

Sheep Sorrel

Rumex Acetosella

Sheep Sorrel or Rumex Acetosella, may also be known as red sorrel, field sorrel and sour weed. It is a species of flowering plant in the buckwheat family. It is a perennial weed. Not native to North America, the plant was introduced from Europe, Asia and the British Isles. One of the common uses of this plant is in foods. The leaves have a tart-lemony flavor. It is a rich source of Vitamin C, E, Beta-Carotene, and other Carotenoids. It has recently received attention for its use in a common cancer tea. A natural anti-oxidant, it has been used to treat a variety of issues from inflammation, diarrhea, scurvy and cancer. Every part of the plant can be used medicinally. The tannins found in this herb may also help to reduce mucus and clear the sinuses. Some other benefits of this plant may be to help enhance the flow of urine, treating kidney and urinary tract diseases, reducing fevers, help to maintain normal levels of blood sugar, intestinal parasites, cooling the liver, strengthening the heart, digestive issues, and as a topical remedy for eczema, herpes, and itchy rashes. You can expect around 0.50$ a pound for this dried herb depending on fluctuating prices and demand.

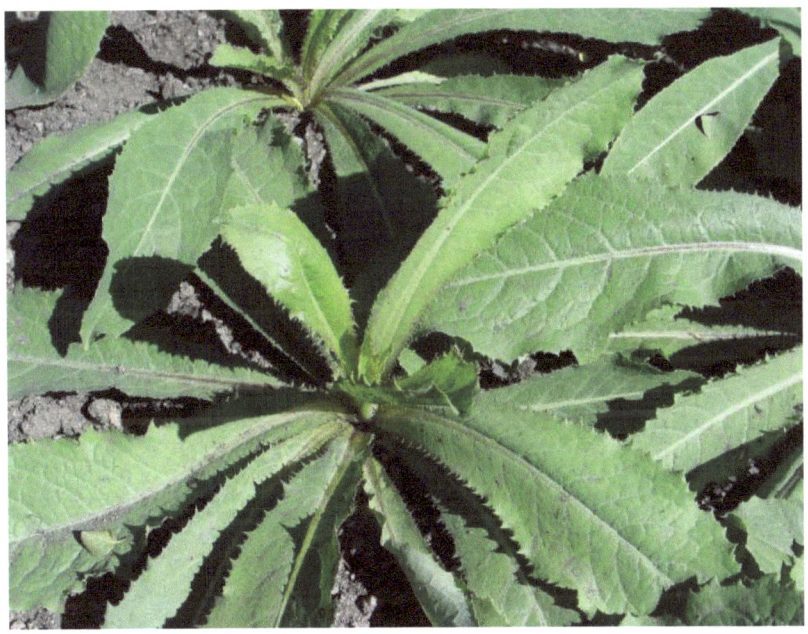

Wild Lettuce Leaf

Lactuca Virosa

Wild Lettuce is very common. It is also known by a great list of names, such as Acrid Lettuce, Bitter Lettuce, German Lactucarium, Green Endive, Lettuce Opium, and Poison Lettuce. Some people are said to inhale wild lettuce for a recreational "high" or hallucinogenic effect. Some of the medicinal uses of this plant include, whooping cough, asthma, urinary tract problems, cough, trouble sleeping, restlessness, excitability in children, painful menstrual periods, excessive sex drive in women, muscular or joint pains, poor circulation, swollen genitals in men, and as an opium substitute in cough medicines. Wild lettuce has calming, relaxing, and pain-relieving effects. When scratched, the plant will secrete a milky, white substance known as lactucarium that can be dried and resembles opium (and has similar effects). You can expect around 0.50$ a pound for this plant.

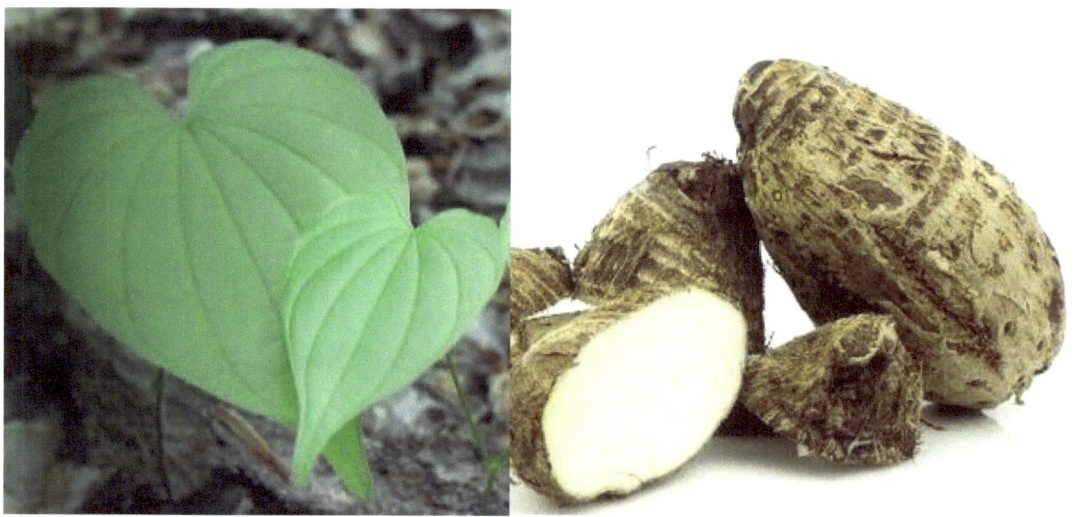

Wild Yam Root

Dioscorea Villosa

Wild Yam Root is native to the eastern part North America. Some of the other names it may be commonly known as depending on where you live are wild yam, colic root, rheumatism root, devil's bones, and four-leaf yam. One of the things it is most known for is its ability to support women in the health of their reproductive systems. It also has powerful antispasmodic and anti-inflammatory properties. It can be used in teas, creams and ointments, or powdered and put into capsules. It is believed to influence hormone balances in a way that can benefit things like morning sickness, premenstrual syndrome, hot flashes, menstrual cramps, vaginal dryness, low libido, and osteoporosis. Wild Yam can be cultivated by harvesting root cuttings to replant in your garden. Root cuttings are generally made in the fall, after the parent plant has matured its fruit and started to die back. After cleaning and drying the roots of this plant, you can expect to gain around 2.00$ a pound from bulk buyers.

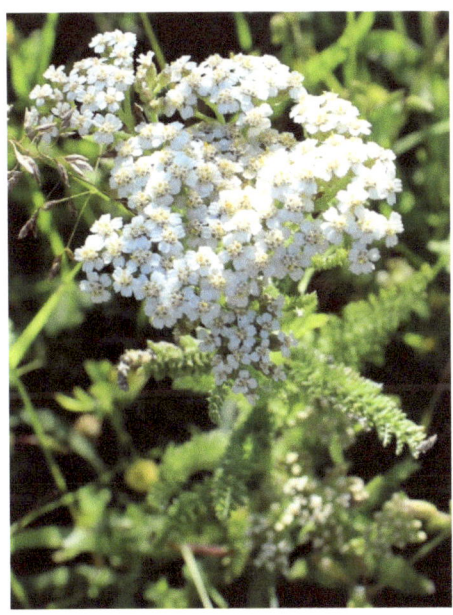

Yarrow Herb

Achillea Millefolium

Yarrow Herb is a flowering plant in the Asteraceae family. Depending on where you live, Yarrow Herb may also be known as thousand-seal, soldier's woundwort, nosebleed plant, old man's pepper, sanguinary, milfoil, thousand-leaf, and devil's nettle. Yarrow is found almost world wide and likes sunny places. It is the parts of the plant that are above ground (or the herbs) that are used medicinally. It has quite a few things that it can be used for. For example, some people chew the fresh leaves of the Yarrow to relieve toothache. Some other things Yarrow is widely used for include fever, hay fever, common cold, loss of appetite, absence of menstruation, diarrhea, dysentery, gastrointestinal tract discomfort, and to induce sweating. Yarrow can be toxic to some animals and humans if mixed with other herbs. As always, use caution if you do not know what you are doing if creating your own home remedies. It is always wise to research your herbs. One can obtain around 0.25$ a pound for the dried herb.

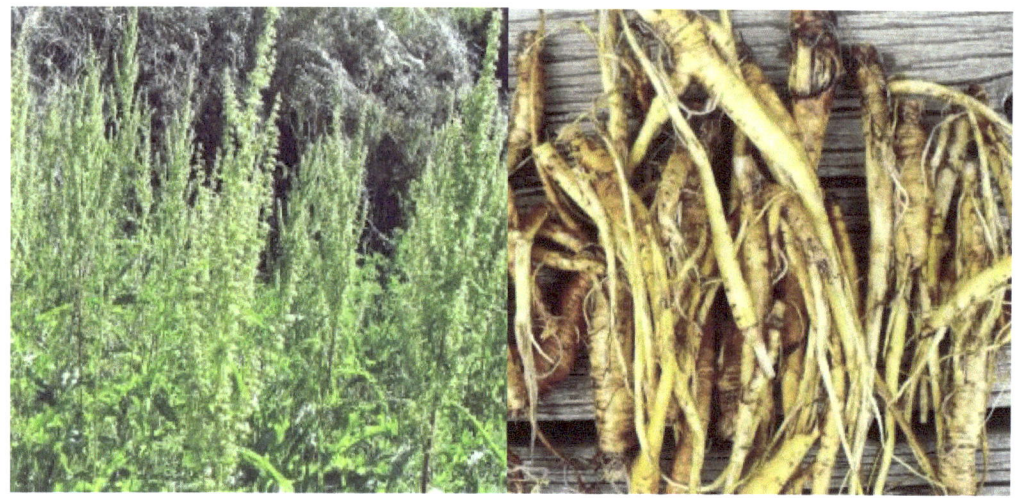

Yellow Dock Herb and Root

Rumex Crispus

Yellow Dock is a perennial flowering plant in the Polygonaceae family. Sometimes known as curly dock or curled dock, it is native to Europe and Asia. It was introduced to North America and has become an invasive species of plant. It can be used eaten as a wild leaf vegetable but the young leaves should be boiled in several changes of water to remove as much of the oxalic acid in the leaves as possible. It can be also added directly to salads in moderate amounts. It can sometimes used to treat anemia because of its high level of iron. Also, it can be made into a poultice to be used on sores, rashes, skin infections, and athlete's foot. The root is harvested in the fall of the year and is traditionally used as a tea or tincture. The herb acts to stimulate peristalsis and increase mucous production and secretion of water in the colon which may help constipation. Some other uses of this plant may include relieve the pain and swelling of nasal passages and the respiratory tract, to treat intestinal infections, fungal infections, and for arthritis. You can expect around 0.50 a pound for the herb and a 1.00$ for the root.

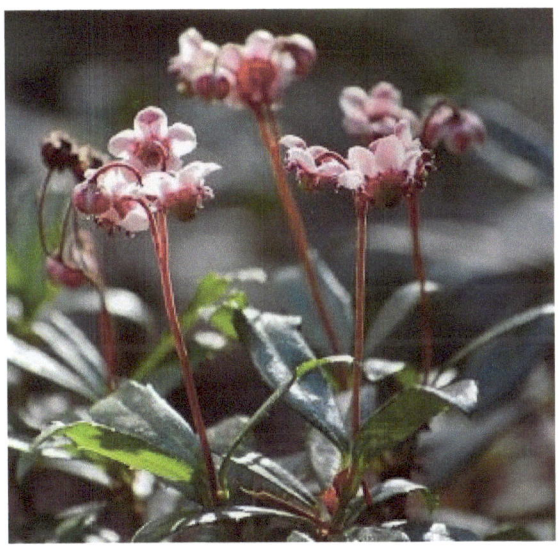

Pipsissewa Herb

Chimaphila Umbellata

Pipsissewa Herb, is a subshrub or that grows back each year from its roots. A subshrub is a perennial plant or small shrub that has a woody base. It is native to much of southern Canada and the northern United States. It was used by Native Americans for its astringent properties. While its leaves are collected in late summer, its scientific name literally means "winter loving". Fresh extract from this herb can be found in cosmetics and lotions but it is usually used by people making home remedies in teas or tinctures. It is sometimes used for flavoring in foods and some apply it directly to the skin for treating sores and blisters. Some of the other things it is widely used for includes teas for urinary tract infections, bladder stones, fluid retention, spasms, epilepsy, anxiety, and cancer. It may help to reduce swelling, be used as an astringent on skin tissues (a drying effect), and kill germs that cause infections in the urinary tract and a variety of other things. Prices can vary from 10.00$ to 40.00$ per pound depending on whether you sell to a bulk buyer or straight to the consumer.

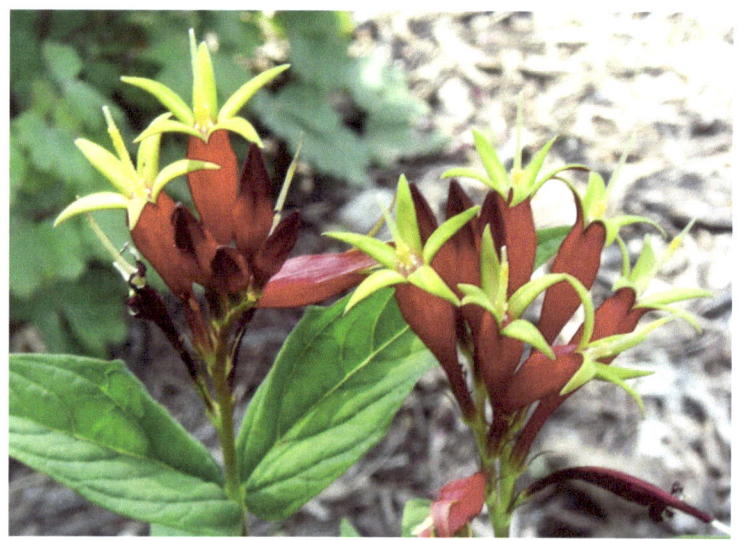

Pink Root

Spigelia Marilandica

Pink Root is an herb but the dried root and bulb are used to make medicine. It can get rid of intestinal worms if taken with a laxative. This method was used in the United States as late as 1955. Some other common names for Pink Root include woodland pinkroot, Indian pink, worm root, wormgrass, star-bloom. It blooms from May to July and is commonly found along the edges of forests in the south Eastern part of the United States. Prices fluctuate so call your local bulk buyer to retrieve a price list but on average you can expect 0.50$ to 1.50$ per pound. You could make more selling straight to the consumer yourself but selling in bulk is usually the best way to go.

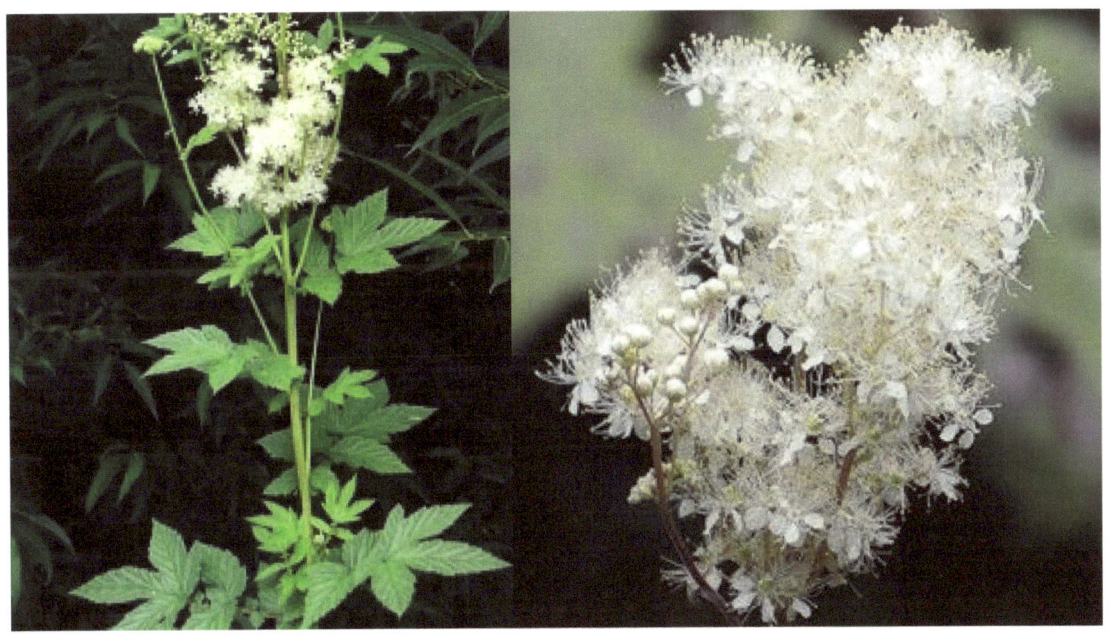

Queen of the Meadow

Filipendula Ulmaria

Queen of the Meadow is a perennial herb in the Rosaceae family. It is commonly found growing in damp meadows and moist places. It is not native to North America but has been introduced and naturalized from Europe and Western Asia. The flower of the plant contains high levels of salicylic acid which is known for its ability to reduce pain. It is one of the compounds used to make aspirin and is used commonly in eczema and psoriasis medicines due to its ability to cause the shedding of the outer layer of skin. It has also been long used as a cure for digestive problems. Some of the other things thins herb may be use for include reducing inflammation and to treat sunburn as well as swelling, arthritis, headaches and coughs. Asthmatics should avoid taking this herb. You can expect anywhere from 2.00$ to 6.00$ per pound of this herb.

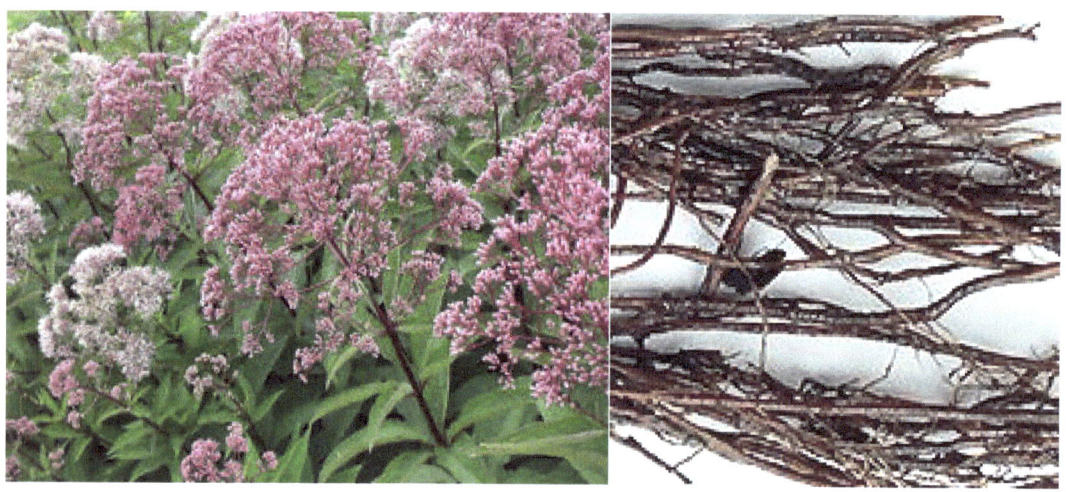

Joe-Pye Root

Eupatorium purpureum

Joe-Pye root is also known as Queen of the Meadow but not the different scientific names and the color of the plants. It is also another plant that is commonly called "Snakeroot". Some of the other names include gravel root, kidney root, mist-flower, purple boneset, eupatorium, trumpet weed, and Sweet Joe-Pye Weed. This perennial herb, found in moist woods and fields throughout Appalachia, is at its height of bloom right now through September. Butterflies are attracted to this plant. It's named after a New England American Indian named Joe Pye, who was said to have cured typhus with it. Native Americans have long used this entire plant in their medicines. The Iroquois and Cherokee used its roots and flowers as a diuretic to help with urinary and kidney ailments, while the roots and leaves could be steeped in hot water and the liquid taken for fever and inflammation. This plant can be dangerous if used without caution. While prices fluctuate you can expect to gain around 2.00$ to 6.00$ for a pound of this root.

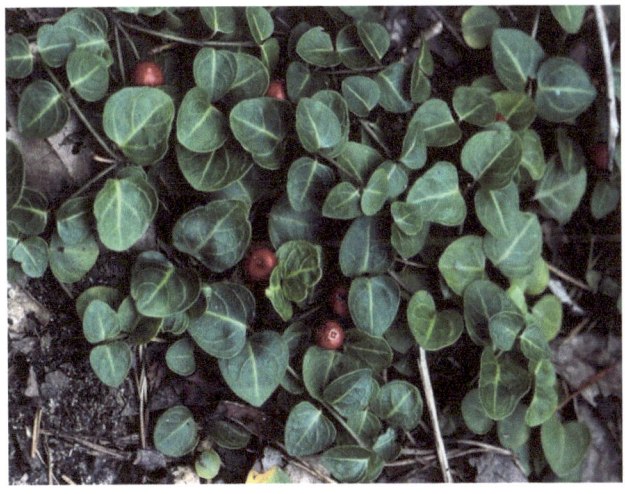

Squaw Vine

Mitchella Repens

Squaw Vine is a perennial herbaceous woody shrub, that is an evergreen with a creeping non climbing vine. Some of the other names it is commonly known as include art-ridge berry, squaw berry, two-eyed berry, running fox, checker berry, deer berry, hill berry, wax cluster, box berry. It is found all over most of the United States and prefers shady areas around trees and shrubs. The above ground parts of the plant are used and should be gathered in the spring or early fall for maximum potency. Native Americans used this herb successfully throughout their entire pregnancies and was taken for weeks before confinement, in order to render parturition safe and easy. It is recommended by herbalists today that it's used only during the last six weeks of pregnancy only because of its slight oxytocic (hastening child birth) properties. It is used in dropsy, suppression of urine, and diarrhea, parturient, diuretic, tonic, astringent. Contact your local buyer to attain the price, but it is powdered and sold to consumers for anywhere between 30.00$ to 90.00$ per pound.

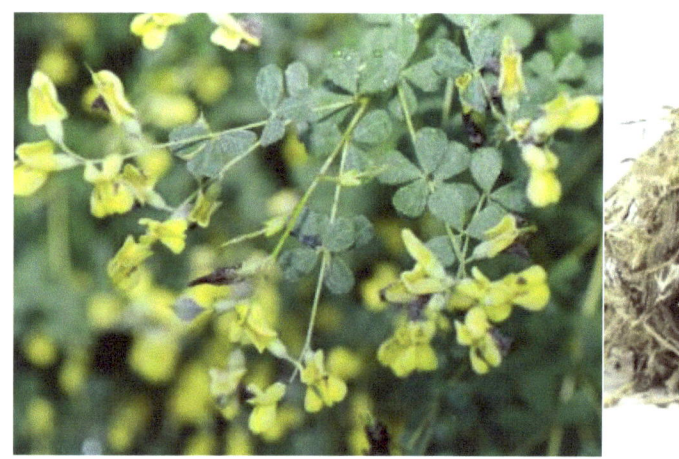 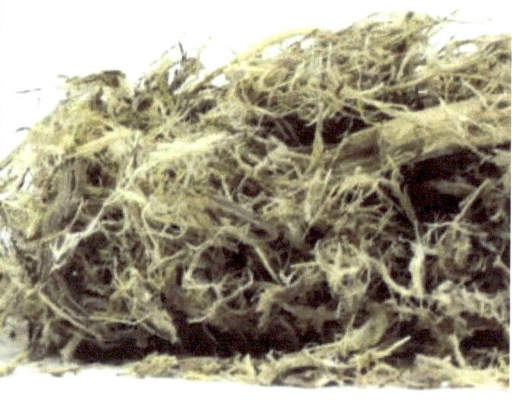

Wild Indigo Root

Baptisia Australis

Wild Indigo is a perennial plant. The flowers can be yellow or purple and are also known as Baptisia root, American indigo, clover bloom, dyer's baptisia, false indigo, horsefly weed, indigo broom, indigo weed, rattle-bush, rattle-weed, yellow broom, yellow indigo. The root is an herb used to make medicines for infections such as diphtheria,

PAGE 51

influenza, swine flu, the common cold and other upper respiratory tract infections, lymph node infections, scarlet fever, malaria, and typhoid. It is native to North America and is very common. It was sometimes used by Native Americans as medicine and it could be made into a dye. It is also sometimes used for sore tonsils, sore throat, swelling of the mouth and throat, fever, boils, and Crohn's disease. It prefers to grow dry soils in woods and clearings, along tree lines, open prairies or hay fields. Contact your buyer to find out the price per pound but it can sell straight to the consumer for anywhere between 50.00$ and 100.00$ per pound.

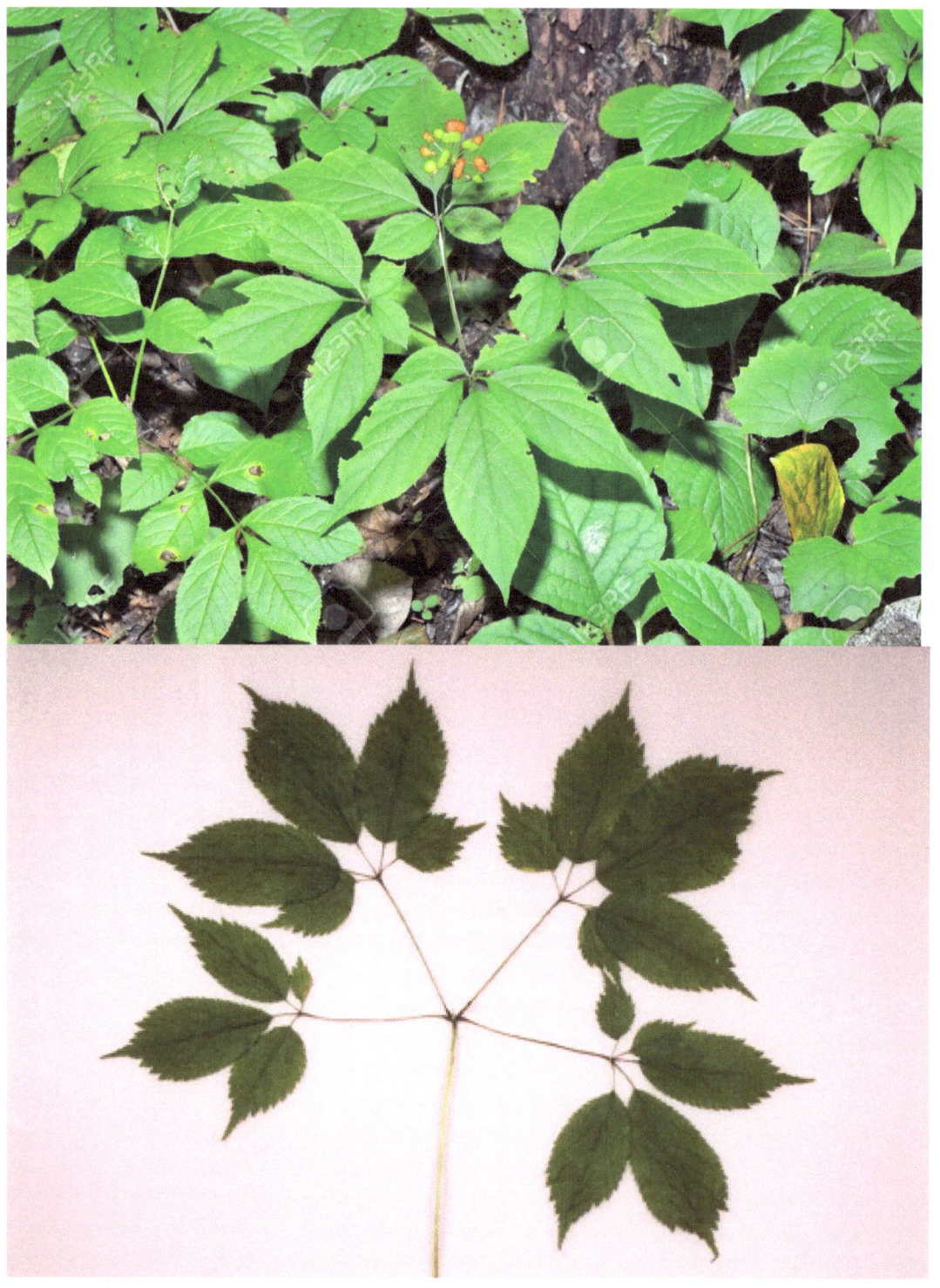

Ginseng

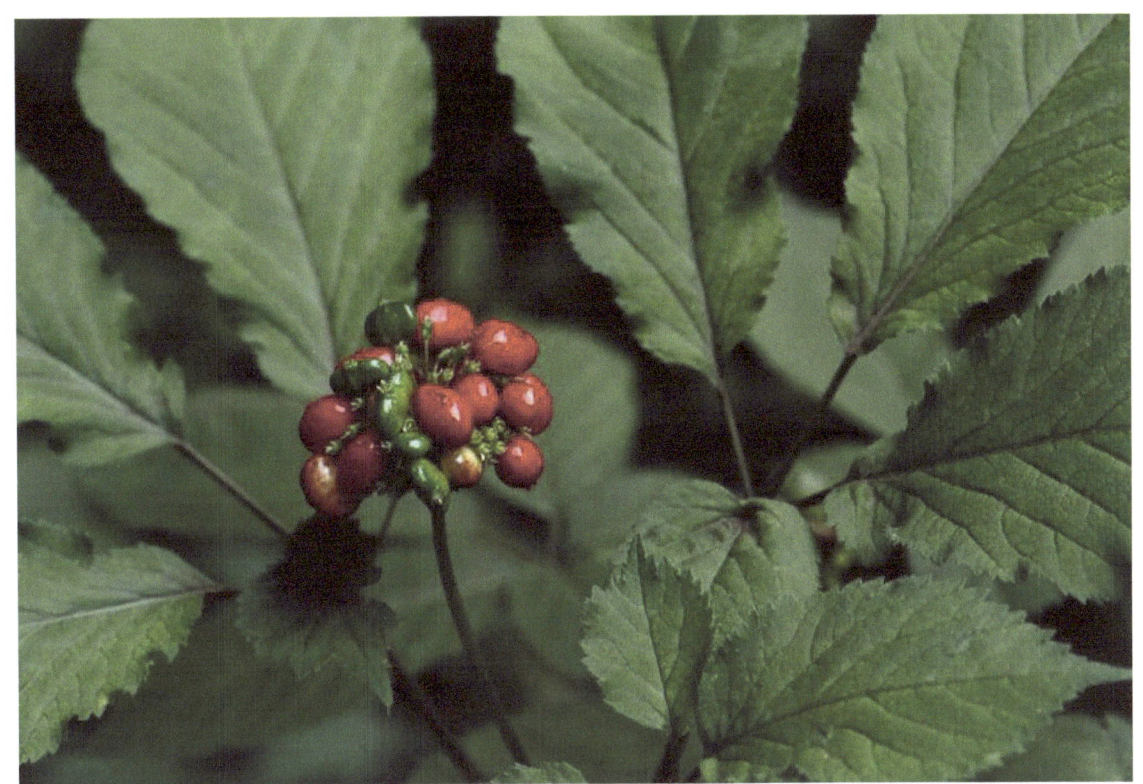

Ginseng

Panax

Ginseng is one of the most sought after and valued roots that you can harvest. Though the prices fluctuate due to time of year, region, and demand, it can sell for anywhere between a 100.00$ to a 1000.00$ per pound. You have to contact your local buyer to get the most current prices. If the price is low, then most people save their harvests, which causes the price to go up. This is true for most roots, herbs, and plants. While ginseng is one of the most if not the most valued root out there, plenty of other things can still command great value.

There are strict rules for harvesting ginseng that I must include. The laws may be different depending on where you live, so be sure to know your local laws concerning the harvesting of ginseng. In nineteen states, ginseng can only be harvested between September 1st and November 30th or December 31st of each year. All other states have laws prohibiting the harvesting of ginseng. Ginseng can generally be classified by how many prongs each plant has. This is also a way to tell the age of the plant. Plants that have fewer than three prongs cannot be harvested by law. The number of prongs a plan has is also a way of determining how prized it is. Generally, the more prongs a plant has, the older the plant is. The older the plant is, the bigger the root is. While ginseng is usually sold by the pound or ounces, roots that are uncommonly large in size can be sold to specialty buyers for higher prices. Ginseng can be one of the hardest plants to find, but I have a few tips that may help you.

Ginseng likes to grow in shady areas in hardwood forests. Train your eyes to look for plants with prongs like shown in the images above. When you see a plant that is pronged like a ginseng plant, the next thing you want to do is take a closer look at the way leaves grow on each prong and the shape of the leaf. There will generally be five leaves per prong.

You will want to look in areas that have a thick growth of trees and shrubs. Look for areas that have a lot of these types of trees. Poplar Trees, Maple Trees, Basswood Trees, Hickory trees, Oak Trees, and Beech Trees. Ginseng grows well in the shade of these trees. A place where people do not generally go will increase your odds greatly.

I have listed other plants in this book that generally grow along with or near ginseng. Blood root is a good plant to look for. It is very common and a lot easier to find. When you find an area that has a lot of blood root, then look around to see if you can find any ginseng. Some other plants that grow well along with or near ginseng include, cohosh, wild yam, goldenseal, may flower, and Solomon's seal.

Ginseng can change as the plant develops and as it grows during the year. We are only interested in mature plants. By mature, I mean plants that have more than three prongs. If the plant is mature, you will see a cluster of whitish green flowers. The flowers will eventually produce red berries. though you will not always see this, it is what you want to look for. When you harvest a plant that has berries, replant the berries in that area after you harvested the plant. This helps to keep ginseng sustainable.

Ginseng can grow in patches or by itself. In most places you will find ginseng, the area will be "hilly". When you find a patch or a plant, look up and down the hill in the area you found the plant. When a plant produces its berries every year, they will fall off or be blown by the wind, or carried by animals usually downhill. Always look both up and down hill from a plant you found to see if there are more.

The plants start producing berries in September, and these berries are the easiest way to find ginseng.

I wanted to include some plants that you can't really sell, but I feel that I should still include. For one simple reason, knowledge. You never know when the day may come that knowing this might just save your life.

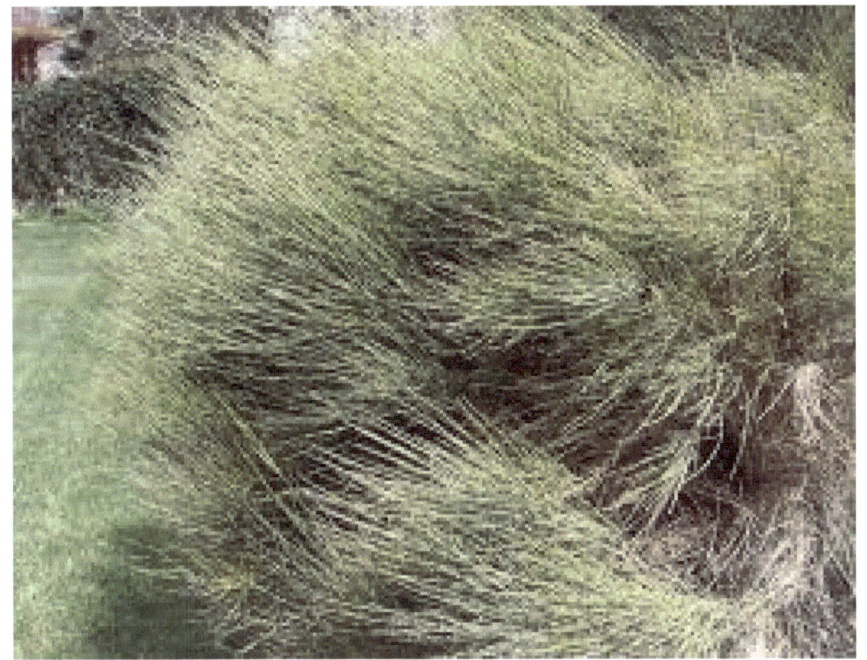

Mormon Tea

Ephedra

Mormon Tea or Ephedra is similar but not to be confused with Ephedrine. Ephedrine is one of the key ingredients on Meth Amphetamines. I am including these just for the knowledge and that you never know when it may be in your benefit to know this stuff. Ephedra is a genus of gymnosperm shrubs. This plant generally grows in the southwestern United States and not in the Appalachian Mountains. There are Ephedrine producing plants that do grow in Appalachia and other places. It is important to note that some of these may be illegal, but they include, Country Mallow, Yellow Horse, Sea Grape, Joint Fir, and Popotillo. I will list some examples of these.

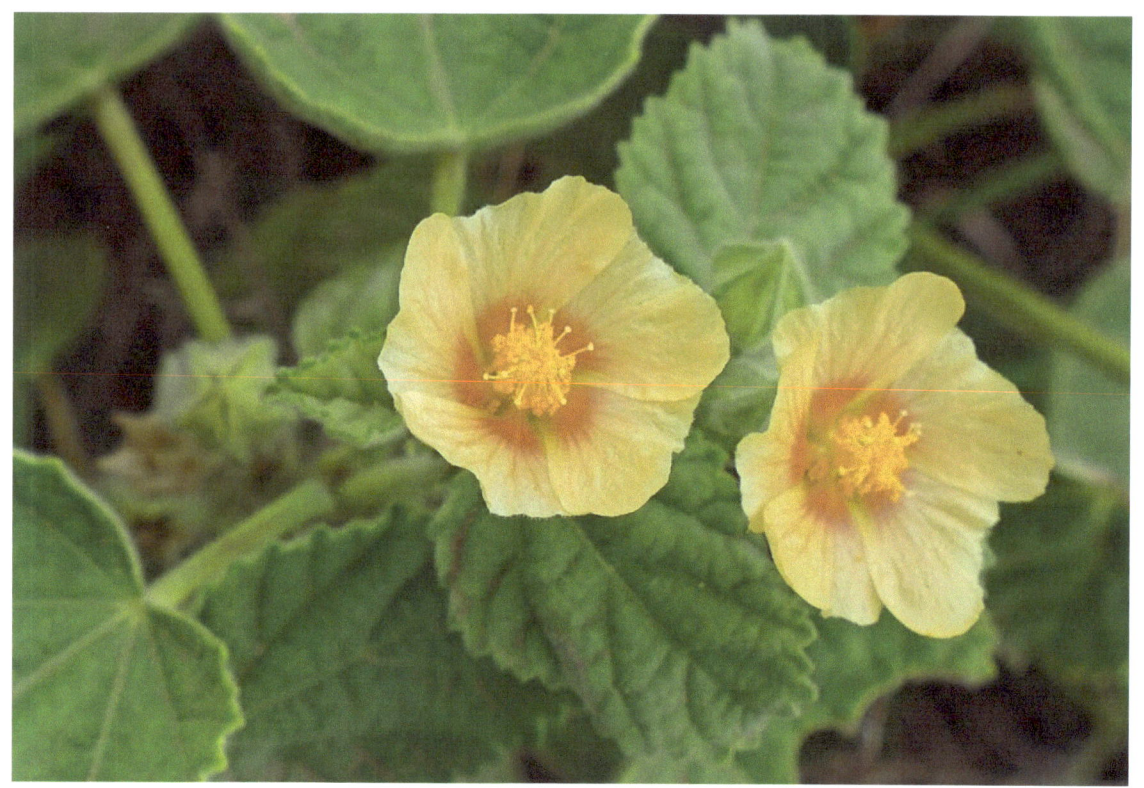

Country Mallow

Sida Cordifolia

Country Mallow is a perennial subshrub of the mallow Malvaceae family native to India. It has naturalized throughout the world, and is considered an invasive weed in Africa, Australia, the southern United States, Hawaiian Islands, New Guinea, and French Polynesia. It is not native to the United States but it a plant that you are likely to run across.

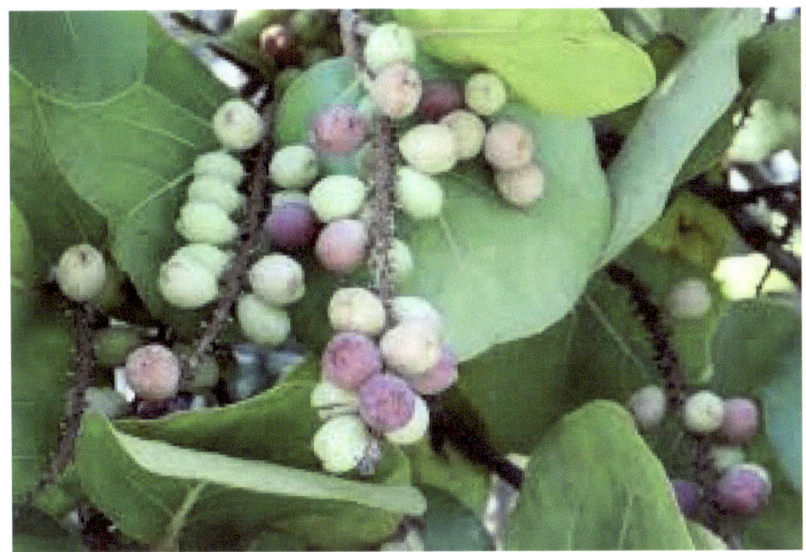

Sea Grape

Coccoloba Uvifera

Sea Grape a species of flowering plant in the buckwheat family. It is native to coastal beaches throughout tropical America and the Caribbean, including southern Florida, the Bahamas.

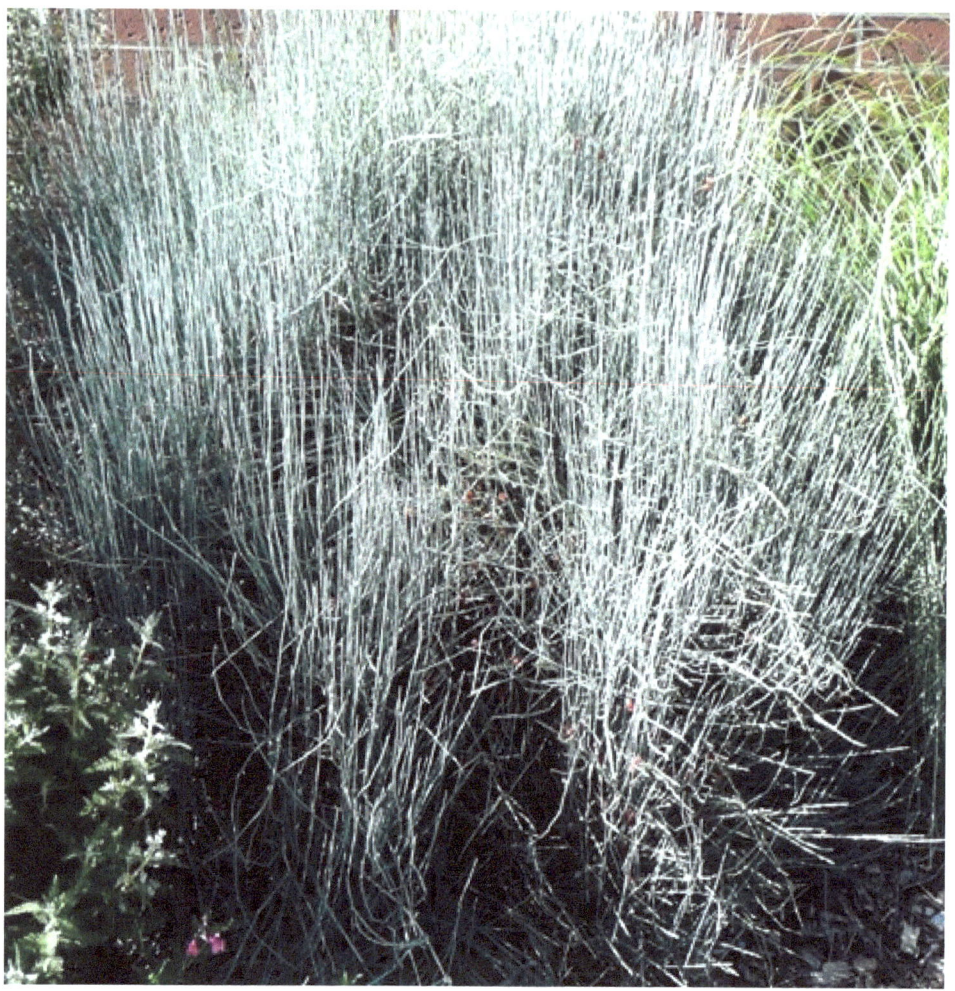

Joint Fir

Ephedra Equisetina

A member of the conifer clan, Ephedra Equisetina is commonly called bluestem joint fir due to its finely textured blue stems. People actually grow this in their gardens. It prefers full sun to partial shade and grows well in, clay, or sandy soil. It can take moderately moist to xeric conditions and is extremely heat and drought tolerant, which makes it a good choice for groupings in difficult areas. It is another plant that grows well in the south western United States.

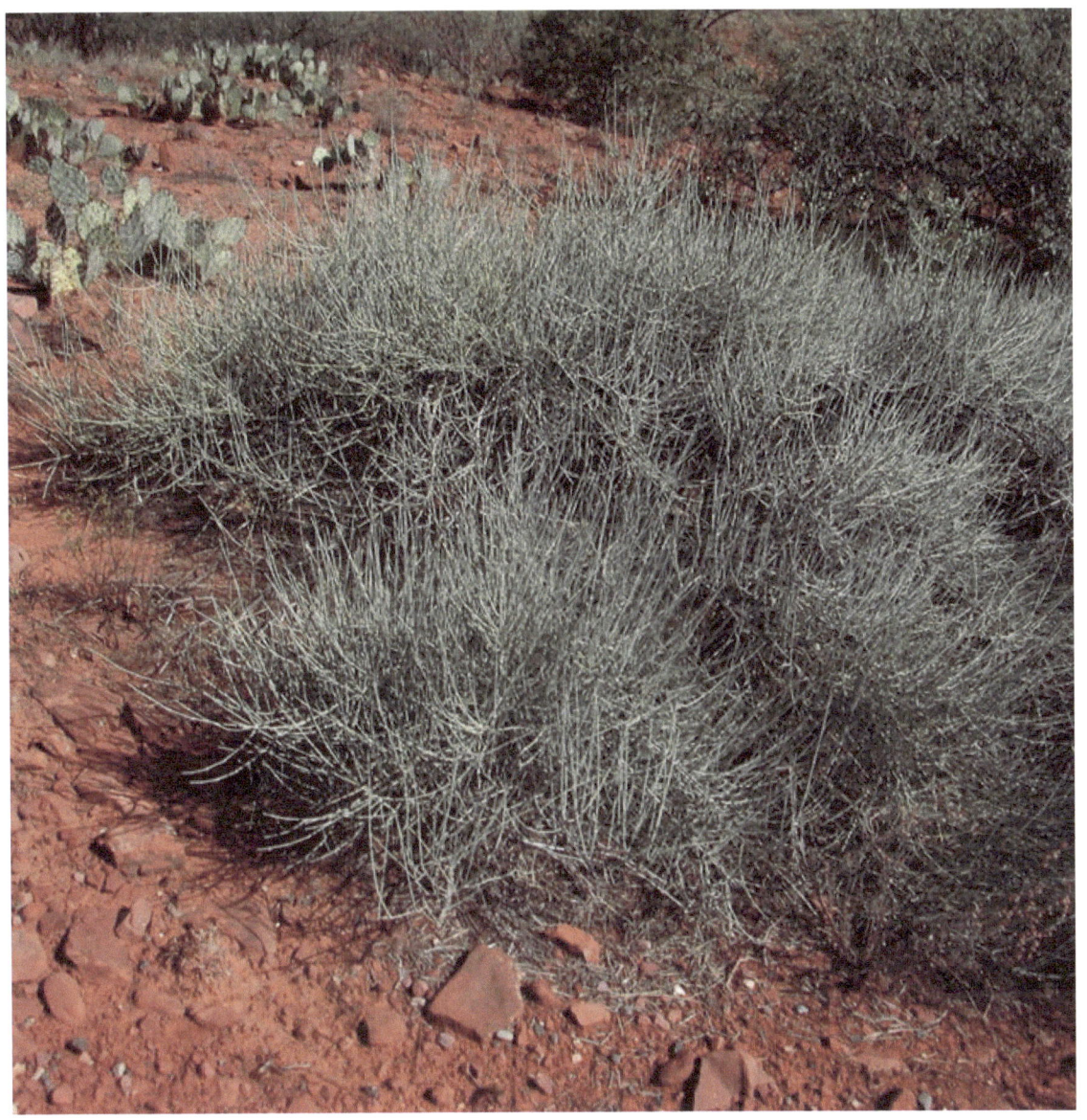

Popotillo

Ephedra Nevadensis

Ephedra Nevadensis is a species of Ephedra native to dry areas of western North

America. It grows west to California and Oregon, east to Texas, and south to Baja

California, including areas of the Great Basin, Colorado Plateau, and the southwest desert

of the United States. There are dozens of these species. I just wanted to include a few.

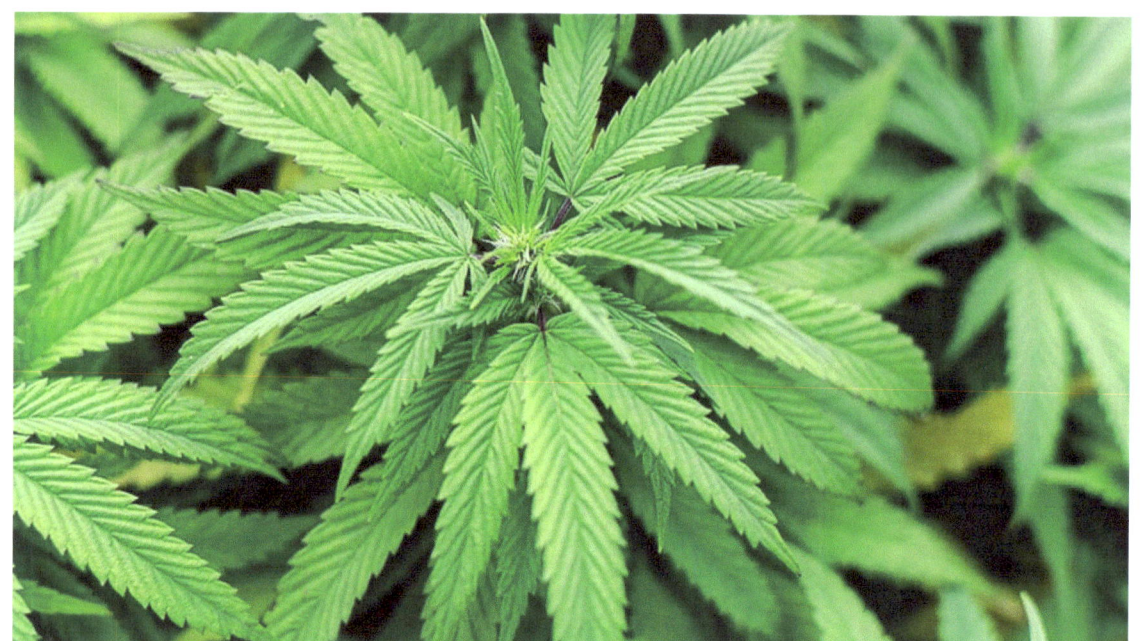

Marijuana

Cannabis

This is the last plant I am including in this particular book. While it is not a plant you can sell (legally) in most states, in some you can and it does grow wild. That is not why I included it. It is a plant that has medicinal use. It was one my Grandmother used from time to time. Currently, the two main cannabinoids from the marijuana plant that are of medical interest are THC and CBD. THC can increase appetite and reduce nausea. THC may also decrease pain, inflammation and muscle control problems. I personally believe it has many more uses for the relief of anxiety and other issues. For years propaganda and misinformation has surrounded this plant. Some were blatant outright lies. One that we were told going through school was that worms would not aerate the soil around the roots of this plant. I did a science project on some of these issues and topics in high-school. To my surprise, they loved it. CBD in marijuana will not get you high and right now studies are being done on some of its medical benefits. The biggest medical benefit is plainly that it will get you high and it is not physically addictive. While I do not smoke marijuana myself (anymore) I am a firm supporter for its legalization of for no other reason than just to bring jobs to areas that need them. Whether it is legal or not, they are still going to grow it. Which brings me to the second biggest reason I included this plant in this book.

When you are out in the wilds harvesting wild herbs, roots, and barks, you may run into dangers. I areas where marijuana is not legal, there are going to be some who still set out traps around their illegal grow sites. While I wish more power to the illegal growers, there is no reason to hurt anyone over it. Sometimes people have been known to trigger their own traps. While marijuana can grow wild, the best thing to do if you are out in the wild and find yourself in the middle of a large patch or marijuana is to,

1. Stop

2. Take a deep breath and look around you.

3. Walk back out taking the exact same steps you took walking in.

This is a very real danger to be aware of. Until the day comes when all the states legalize this plant, it always will be. I hope to later write a book on plants such as this, just for the sake of knowledge.

Here is a list of other things that you can collect and harvest in the wild for money or home remedies. Some of these are actually worth quite a bit of money while others not so much, but all can bring you an extra source of income.

Agarikon (Fomitopsis officinalis)

Alder (Alnus rubra)

Ambrosia (Ambrosia chamissonis)

Anemone (Pulsatilla occidentalis)

Arugula (Eruca vesicaria ssp. Sativa)

Arnica (Arnica cordifolia/tomentella)

Artist's Conk (Ganoderma applanatum)

Ashwaganda (Withania somniferum)

Aspen (Populus tremuloides)

Balsamroot (Balsamorhiza saggitata)

Baneberry (Actea rubra)

Bayberry (Myrica californica)

Beebalm (Monarda didyma)

Betony (Stachys officinalis)

Bilberry (Vaccinium myrtillus)

Bittersweet (Solanum dulcamara)

Blackberries (Rubus armeniacus)

Blackroot (Veronicastrum virginicum)

Blessed Thistle (Cnicus benedictus)

Bleeding Heart (Dicentra formosa)

Burdock (Arctium lappa)

Bugleweed (Lycopus americanus)

Butterbur (Petasites palmatus)

Calamus, American (Acorus calamus)

Calendula (Calendula officinalis)

California Bay (Umbellularia californica)

California Poppy (Eschscholzia californica)

Cascara Sagrada (Frangula purshiana)

Catnip (Nepeta cataria)

Cedar, Incense (Calocedrus decurrens)

Cedar, Western Red (Thuja plicata)

Celandine (Chelidonium majus)

Chickweed (Stellaria media)

Cleavers (Galium aparine)

Corn Lily (Veratrum californicum)

Cow Parsnip (Heracleum lanatum)

Cottonwood (Populus trichocarpa)

Dandelion (Taraxacum officinale)

Devil's Club (Oplopanax horridus)

Dogbane, Spreading (A. androsaemifolium)

Elderberry (Sambucus caerulea)

Elderflower (Sambucus caerulea)

Elecampane (Inula helenium)

Epazote (Chenopodium ambrosioides)

Fireweed (Epilobium angustifolia)

Feverfew (Tanacetum parthenium)

Fireweed (Epilobium angustifolia)

Goldenrod (Solidago canadensis)

Gotu Kola (Centella asiatica)

Gromwell (Lithospermum ruderale)

Gumweed (Grindelia squarrosa)

Hawthorn (Crataegus douglasii)

Holy Basil (Ocimum sanctum)

Horsechestnut (Aesculus hippocastanum)

Horsetail (Equisetum telmateia)

Hops (Humulus lupulus)

Horseradish (Armoracia rusticana)

Hyssop (Hyssopus officinalis)

Iknish (Lomatium californicum)

Indian Warrior (Pedicularis densiflora)

Inside-Out Flower (Vancouveria hexandra)

Japanese Knotweed (Polygonum cuspidatum)

Joe-Pye Weed, Gravelroot (Eupatorium purpureum)

Kinnikinnik (Arctostaphylos uva-ursi)

Larch, Western (Larix occidentalis)

Lavender (Lavandula angustifolia)

Lemon Balm (Melissa officinalis)

Licorice Fern (Polypodium glycyrrhiza)

Lobelia (Lobelia inflata)

Lomatium (Lomatium dissectum)

Lungwort (Lobaria pulmonaria)

Madrone (Arbutus menziesii)

Manzanita (Arctostaphylos viscida)

Marshmallow (Althaea officinalis)

Meadowsweet (Filipendula ulmaria)

Melilot (Melilotus alba)

Mugwort (Artemisia douglasiana)

Nettle (Urtica dioica)

Oats, Milky (Avena sativa)

Oatstraw (Avena sativa)

Oregon Grape, Low (Mahonia nervosa)

Oregon Grape, Tall (Mahonia aquifolium)

Orris Root (Iris florentina)

Osha (Ligusticum canbyii)

Pearly Everlasting (Anaphalis margaritacea)

Peppermint (Mentha piperita)

Periwinkle (Vinca major)

Plantain, Lance Leaf (Plantago lanceolata)

Raspberry (Rubus idaeus)

Red-Belted Polypore (Fomitopsis pinicola)

Red Clover (Trifolium pratense)

Red Osier Dogwood (Cornus sericea)

Reishi, Oregon (Ganoderma oregonense)

Rose (Rosa gymnocarpa)

Rue (Ruta graveolens)

Salal (Gaultheria shallon)

Sage (Salvia officinalis)

Sarsaparilla (Aralia nudicaulis)

Scotch Broom (Cytisus scoparius)

Self-Heal (Prunella vulgaris)

Silk Tassel (Garrya fremontii)

Skullcap (Scutellaria lateriflora)

Soaproot (Chlorogalum pomeridianum)

Spikenard (Aralia californica)

Spikenard (Aralia californica)

Spilanthes (Spilanthes acmella)

Spruce, Sitka (Picea sitchensis)

St. John's Wort (Hypericum perforatum)

Stevia (Stevia rebaudiana)

Sweet Annie (Artemisia annua)

Sweet Flag (Acorus calamus)

Sweet Root (Osmorrhiza occidentalis)

Sweet Clover (Melilotus albus)

Tansy Ragwort (Senecio jacobaea)

Teasel (Dipsacus sylvestris)

Thyme (Thymus vulgaris)

Turkey Tail (Trametes versicolor)

Usnea (Usnea spp.)

Valerian, Sitka (Valeriana sitchensis)

Vervain, Blue (Verbena hastata)

Wild Carrot Seed (Daucus carota)

Western Red Cedar (Thuja plicata)

Winter Savory (Satureja montana)

Wormwood (Artemisia absinthium)

Yellow Pond Lily (Nuphar polysepalum)

Yerba Mansa (Anemopsis californica)

Yerba Santa (Eriodictyon californicum)

Yew (Taxus brevifolia)

In Memory of Ruby Campbell, Irene Clemons, and Joan Williams.

I never told you all how much I appreciate the time and effort you gave me and the things you taught me. The most valuable thing we have in this world is time and none of us truly appreciate it............. Until we are about to run out of it.

www.ingramcontent.com/pod-product-compliance
Lightning Source LLC
Chambersburg PA
CBHW041314180526
45172CB00004B/1099